LECTURE NOTES ON CLINICAL MEDICINE AND SURGERY FOR DENTAL STUDENTS

LECTURE NOTES ON
CLINICAL MEDICINE AND SURGERY
FOR DENTAL STUDENTS

Edited by
D. Maclean
MB, ChB, PhD, FRCP
Department of Pharmacology and Clinical
Pharmacology, University of Dundee

P. E. Preece
MD, FRCS
Department of Surgery
University of Dundee

THIRD EDITION

Blackwell Scientific Publications
Oxford London Edinburgh
Boston Palo Alto Melbourne

© 1972, 1977, 1986 by
Blackwell Scientific Publications
Editorial offices:
Osney Mead, Oxford, OX2 0EL
8 John Street, London, WC1N 2ES
23 Ainslie Place, Edinburgh, EH3 6AJ
52 Beacon Street, Boston
    Massachusetts 02108, USA
667 Lytton Avenue, Palo Alto
    California 94301, USA
107 Barry Street, Carlton
    Victoria 3053, Australia

First published 1972
Second edition 1977
Reprinted 1979
Third edition 1986

DISTRIBUTORS
USA
    Blackwell Mosby Book Distributors
    11830 Westline Industrial Drive
    St Louis, Missouri 63141

Canada
    Blackwell Mosby Book Distributors
    120 Melford Drive, Scarborough
    Ontario M1B 2X4

Australia
    Blackwell Scientific Publications
        (Australia) Pty Ltd
    107 Barry Street
    Carlton, Victoria 3053

British Library
Cataloguing in Publication Data

Lecture notes on medicine and surgery for
    dental students.—3rd ed.
    1. Pathology   2. Wounds and
                         injuries
    I. Maclean, D.   II. Preece, P.E.
    616'.00246176   RB111

    ISBN 0-632-01114-9

Typeset by Pennart Typesetting
(Edinburgh) Ltd, and printed and bound
in Great Britain by Billings and Sons
Ltd, London, Oxford, Worcester.

Contents

Contributors

All from the University of Dundee
and the Dundee teaching hospitals

C. B. Ballinger BSc, MRCP, FRCPsych, Consultant Psychiatrist.
E. M. Brookes FRCPath, Regional Director, East of Scotland Blood Transfusion Service.
R. A. Clark BSc, FRCP, Consultant Physician.
R. S. Clark MRCP, Lecturer in Medicine.
P. G. Davey MD, MRCP, Senior Registrar in Communicable Diseases.
D. L. W. Davidson BSc (Hons), FRCP (Edin), Consultant Neurologist.
A. L. Forrest FFARCS, Consultant Anaesthetist.
N. A. Irvine BSc, MRCP, Lecturer in Clinical Pharmacology.
P. B. James MB, ChB, DIH, PhD, MFOM, Senior Lecturer in Occupational Medicine.
I. W. W. Jeffrey PhD, FDS, LDSRCS (Edin), Senior Lecturer in Conservative Dentistry.
R. T. Jung MA, MD, FRCP Consultant Physician.
M. R. Kerr FRCP (Edin), Consultant in Communicable Diseases.
T. Lakshmipathi MB, BS (Madras), Associate Specialist in Dermatology.
D. G. McDevitt DSc, MD, FRCP, Professor of Clinical Pharmacology.
D. Maclean PhD, FRCP, Senior Lecturer in Pharmacology and Therapeutics.
W. J. MacLennan MD, FRCP, Reader in Geriatric Medicine.
R. W. Newton FRCP (Edin), Consultant Physician.
D. Parratt MD, FRCPath, Senior Lecturer in Medical Microbiology.
N. Patel MRCOG, Consultant Obstetrician.
C. R. Paterson MA, DM, BSc, FRCPath, Senior Lecturer in Biochemical Medicine.
C. R. Pennington BSc, MD, FRCP (Edin), Consultant Physician.

P. E. Preece MD, FRCS, Senior Lecturer in Surgery.

A. C. Scott MD, FRCPath, Senior Lecturer in Medical Microbiology.

J. S. Scott FRCR, FFR, DMTR, Director, Tayside Area Radiotherapy and Oncology Service.

N. H. Smith MRCGP, General Practitioner.

W. K. Stewart MD, PhD, FRCP, Senior Lecturer in Medicine.

G. R. Tudhope BSc, MD, FRCP, Reader in Therapeutics.

M. Wilkinson MD, FRCP, Consultant Physician.

R. A. Yorston MB, ChB, Associate Specialist in Otolaryngology (now retired).

Preface

The many recent advances in medical science make a new edition of this book essential. This differs from previous editions in that now each chapter has been contributed by an author who is currently practising in the field covered. Dr Peter M. Ford is succeeded as co-editor with Dr Derek Maclean by Mr Paul E. Preece.

The content of the curriculum for training of health care professionals has to change constantly in response to both the changing needs of the community being served and the continual advance in knowledge. The aspiring Bachelor of Dental Surgery, confronted by the need to learn Medicine and Surgery as but a small part of the undergraduate course, might be forgiven for wondering if society would not be better training its dentists as medical practitioners first! Realistically, dental students must study a distillate of Medicine and Surgery.

A consensus of what this should be in the UK was agreed in 1981 at a conference of those who teach these subjects to dental students. A summary of this was published in the *Lancet* in 1982.* It is on the basis of these recommendations, to which the editors subscribed as participants at the conference, that this book has been compiled. Teaching in Medicine and Surgery is intended to broaden the basis of the professional education of dentists, helping them to understand new advances and to encourage continued learning. It is also of value in dental practice, where it should ensure the safety of patients and staff, recognition of high-risk subjects, good patient relations, with understanding of clinical phenomena, and the ability to cope with emergencies. The student's clinical judgment will be improved as will his ability to communicate effectively with other health care professionals, in particular to recognize where there is an indication for a second opinion and understand the principles of the maintenance of health. A sound knowledge of Medicine and Surgery also equips the dentist for career diversification, in teaching, research, preventive medicine, as well as in day to day clinical practice.

Sections have been written to stand on their own. We have intentionally omitted detailed accounts of areas which we know to be taught in detail in the dental curriculum.

*Medical Teaching of Dental Students. *Lancet*, 1982,i,332. The full report is available from the Nuffield Foundation, Nuffield Lodge, Regents Park, London NW1.

ACKNOWLEGEMENTS

The editors have been greatly assisted by Dr Ian W. M. Jeffrey and his colleagues at Dundee Dental School who have read through the text to check clarity and relevance to dental students. Dr George Tudhope has made an overview of the whole text for consistency.

1 History, examination and precautions

History taking
The dentist/patient relationship begins with history taking. This consists of:
    present symptoms,
    current drug treatment,
    past illness and operations and their sequelae,
    health and illnesses of relatives,
    occupation and pastimes.

Any patient may have the unacceptable or the unexpected in his background. Be alert, be suspicious and be prepared to elicit information not readily volunteered by the patient, e.g. a patient with abnormal bleeding of the gums may have leukaemia; a past history of rheumatic fever predisposes to the risk of subacute bacterial endocarditis. Unrecognized venereal disease is a danger to both the patient and the dentist.

Physical examination
The extent of the physical examination varies. It is influenced by:
    symptoms of the patient,
    setting of the consultation,
    specialty of the clinician.

For the dentist, valuable information about general health is to be had from observation of exposed parts:
1. *General*:
    nutrition,
    respiration,
    responsiveness.
2. *Skin*:
    colour (pallor, cyanosis, jaundice),
    texture (sweaty, scaly).

3. *Facies*:
   thin and drawn,
   round and plethoric.
4. *Lips*:
   discoloured, cracked or ulcerated.
5. *Hands*:
   colour,
   clubbing,
   arthropathy.
6. *Nails*:
   cyanosed,
   flattened,
   infected.

The detection of signs previously unnoticed necessitates referral for elucidation of their precise cause.

Precautions: principles of prevention: prophylaxis
'Prevention is better than cure.'

Increasingly, clinical practice is capable of implementing this old cliché. To do so requires active consideration of all the possible complications of a given treatment before it is started. Prevention of the following apply particularly in surgery:

Bleeding (congenital, liver function, vitamin K, platelets);
Coma (diabetes, liver disease, nervous system, vascular);
Infection (incision, chest, systemic, e.g. tetanus);
Renal failure (adequate fluids, monitoring output);
Thromboembolism (dextran, heparin, mobilization);
Wound dehiscence (incisions, nutrition, suture materials).

Bleeding
Before causing any bleeding, ensure that it will stop. From the history, rule out anticoagulant therapy or any abnormal bleeding tendency. The coumarin drugs, particularly warfarin, are the most widely used anticoagulants, being less likely to cause sensitivity reactions than phenindione. Oral anticoagulant therapy is monitored by means of measurement of the *prothrombin time* or *thrombotest*. Treatment with other drugs affects the tendency to bleed in these patients, e.g. ingestion of aspirin is liable to cause haemorrhage, from inhibition of thromboxane synthesis, impaired platelet aggregation or reduced hepatic synthesis of clotting factors. Withdrawal of anticonvulsants in

patients who have been maintained on these in addition to oral antico-agulants similarly may cause haemorrhage because of the withdrawal of induction of the enzymes that normally metabolize warfarin. Some drugs, such as aspirin and dipyridamole, reduce platelet adhesiveness. They are used to reduce the tendency to thrombus formation in arteries. They can, however, also lead to increased blood loss at op-eration.

Haemophilia A is the most common of the potentially severe in-herited bleeding disorders. Surgical procedures on patients so affected do not always require Factor VIII infusion (p.83). In practice, occa-sionally when bleeding is a problem in a surgical procedure, a diagnosis of *Christmas disease* is made where the inherited deficiency is that of Factor IX. Although not congenital, a deficiency of platelet num-bers is called *thrombocytopenia*. The platelet precursors are present but they give rise to insufficient platelets. Clot retraction is impaired and the capillary fragility test is positive. The clotting time is normal, but the bleeding time is prolonged, making surgery without platelet supplementation dangerous.

Blood clotting is dependent on normal function of the liver which synthesizes prothrombin and Factors VII and X from the fat-soluble vitamin K, the absorption of which requires bile salts. These are pre-vented from entering the bowel in obstructive jaundice, a condition where parenteral vitamin K therapy is essential *before* surgery is per-formed.

Certain drugs are used to facilitate blood clotting. Aminocaproic acid and tranexamic acid work by inhibiting plasminogen activation and so interfere with fibrinolysis. They therefore have a role in den-tal extraction in haemophiliacs (p.84).

Coma

Cerebral function can be affected by surgical procedures. The com-monest problem in practice is the vasovagal attack, which can occur in any patient anticipating or being submitted to even very minor pro-cedures such as venepuncture. Prophylaxis of harm from this is achieved by ensuring that patients are supine before any procedure is performed. In such a position, adequate cerebral blood flow can be maintained.

Diabetic patients require special consideration when undergoing surgery. The greatest danger from which known diabetics are at risk is peri-operative *hypoglycaemia* during operation under general an-aesthesia. Modern diabetic management involves giving the insulin as usual and controlling its hypoglycaemic effect with i.v. dextrose under blood glucose monitoring. Ketoacidosis is only likely to occur in previously unrecognized diabetics and can be prevented by the simple measure of always testing the urine for sugar before surgery.

Liver disease can impair the ability to metabolize drugs, including both local or general anaesthetics, and should be excluded before these are administered. Drugs given for their effects on the nervous system, particularly some psychotropic drugs and anticonvulsants, can interact adversely with analgesics and anaesthetics, predisposing to coma, either by direct action on the brain or by indirect action by suppressing respiration.

Infection

The prevention of infection in surgical practice is fundamental. It is most conveniently subdivided into prevention of general (systemic) infection and local, i.e. confined to the site of operation. The whole gamut of aseptic technique, including the use of operating theatres, the wearing of special garments including masks and gloves, sterilization of instruments and antiseptic preparation of the operation site, is designed to minimize the risk of infection and its sequelae. All such measures, when effective, prevent local sepsis and thereby also systemic spread. Some specific measures are required, however, to prevent systemic infections or complications, e.g. patients sustaining contaminated (usually accidental) wounds must receive immunization against tetanus. Infection with this disease, followed by recovery, does not impart lifelong immunity. Systemic sequelae can ensue in operating on patients who have damaged heart valves or implanted prostheses. Such operations require systemic antibiotics to be given before surgery begins. Pre- and post-operative physiotherapy can help to prevent post-operative chest infections.

The prevention of local infection is facilitated by placing the incision in the line of the natural creases because this encourages faster healing. The scar is also less prominent. Tissue should be handled as gently as possible. Sutures should be as fine as possible and should just approximate the edges without being too tight.

Renal failure

In addition to their function in effecting water and electrolyte balance, the kidneys have a role in metabolizing drugs, especially analgesics. Before surgery it is essential to know that a patient has normal or at least adequate renal function, the simplest test for which is measurement of the serum urea and creatinine levels. During and after surgery, adequate urine output must be observed, with regular checks on the quantity of the urine passed. For prolonged surgical procedures, this necessitates the passage of a urethral catheter, which can be connected to a urinometer by means of which the volume of urine passed per unit time, e.g. per hour, can be checked. The specific gravity taken with repeat serum urea or creatinine measurements gives a simple guide to the concentrating power of the kidneys. For adequate renal function to be maintained, the surgeon must ensure that adequate fluids are given, the intravenous route being essential for these where patients have to be fasted. The prescription of fluids has to take account of not only volume and electrolyte requirements but also the balance between crystalloid (i.e. ionized salts like sodium chloride) and colloid (i.e. larger particles like albumin). These prescriptions require consideration of cardiovascular and pulmonary factors, such as whether the patient has a tendency to heart failure (as after myocardial infarction) or to bronchospasm (as in an asthmatic).

Thromboembolism (p.69)
One of the most terrible complications of surgery is the formation of a blood clot which then migrates to the lung where it occludes a major pulmonary vessel and so causes sudden death. This occurs after major surgery, i.e. operations on the abdomen or pelvis, and after surgery to the hip where the operation is adjacent to the large iliac veins. The risk is increased in patients who have been immobile prior to surgery, in the obese and in patients with malignant diseases. Agents are available which, if given over the operative period, significantly reduce the risk of deep vein thrombosis and pulmonary embolism. The macromolecular substance dextran (particularly dextran 70) lowers blood viscosity when given intravenously. To achieve this it expands the blood volume. Heparin is given for this purpose in low dose (5000 units) by subcutaneous injection, pre-operatively and then 8 or 12 hourly until the patient is ambulant. Both agents tend to increase the likelihood of peri-operative bleeding, but this disadvantage is far outweighed by the reduced risk of fatal thromboembolism.

Wound dehiscence
Separation of a wound, primarily closed at the time of operation, is a setback for both patient and surgeon. It is alarming, increases the risk of infection, predisposes to hernia formation, leaves an ugly scar, and

can necessitate another anaesthetic, with its attendant risks. Several of the factors which minimize infection after surgery also contribute to preventing wound dehiscence. These include:

Aseptic technique,
Antiseptic preparation of operation site,
Clean-cut incision in a skin crease,
Meticulous haemostasis,
Fine suture materials just approximating the tissue without compression or tension.

Where is it is difficult to obtain a good state of nutrition pre-operatively, parenteral feeding and dietary supplementation with vitamin C and zinc preparations, which are essential for wound healing, can prevent this problem.

2 First aid, emergency management and trauma

The objective of first aid is the maintenance of adequate cerebral oxygenation and the prevention of incidental damage, while normal self-preservation is impaired or impossible. The commonest situations where first aid is required are: collapse, haemorrhage, injury and post-operative care.

First aid involves attending to
Airway,
Circulation,
Nervous system,
Systemic effects of injury.

Airway
Respiratory embarrassment can be caused by:
1. *Obstruction*,
2. *Inhalation*,
3. *Paralysis*,
4. *Trauma*.
1. In unconsciousness, particularly if the subject is supine, the tongue falls posteriorly, occluding the airway. This can be prevented by having the patient lying on his or her side, with the head dependent, with the angles of the mandibles drawn firmly forward. Oedema glottidis, as part of an acute allergic reaction, can obstruct the pharynx, and oedema or spasm of the vocal cords can obstruct the larynx. Foreign bodies can occlude any part of the lumen of the respiratory tract, which can also be obstructed suddenly by extrinsic means such as trauma or haemorrhage into an adjacent tumour.

   A first-aid method for attempting to clear the airway into which a foreign body has been inhaled is known as the *Heimlich manoeuvre*. The patient lies with the head dependent. The rib cage is surrounded by the arms of the assistant who compresses this

7

forcefully, to expel the foreign body. The system is controversial since it may cause damage to the liver or the ribs and lungs. Nevertheless, in an emergency situation, where no skilled help or special equipment is available, it can save life.

Liquids, either extrinsic to the respiratory system, such as inhaled water or blood, or intrinsic, such as secretions from the respiratory tract itself, can effectively cause death by drowning. This is preventable by posture, aided by suction. Postural drainage can be specially effectively done by a physiotherapist and a flexible bronchoscope can be used to unplug distal parts of the bronchial tree, such as in lobar collapse.

2. In addition to the obstructive effects of inhalation, whether this be by foreign bodies or liquids, irritant substances can be inhaled, particularly gastric secretions, vegetable products, e.g. peanut, and toxic gases from fires. These induce an intense, acute inflammatory response within the entire bronchial tree, which rapidly impairs gaseous exchange, and can readily cause irreversible damage to the affected lung. If such irritation is suspected, in addition to mechanical removal of aspirated and inspired material, powerful anti-inflammatory drugs are given, particularly high doses of corticosteroids. Some inhaled gases, e.g. carbon monoxide, poison haemoglobin or the gas transport enzymes, a process which is irreversible.

3. Paralysis of the respiratory system occurs either within the central nervous system or peripherally. Trauma, infection and drugs can cause this, e.g. head injury, poliomyelitis and muscle relaxants respectively.

4. The effects of injury can be *direct* or *indirect*, e.g. division of the phrenic nerve (the fourth cervical nerve) immobilizes the hemidiaphragm which it supplies, limiting voluntary respiration and respiratory excursion. Fracture of a single rib can lead to puncture of the pleura and lung, which tends to collapse, sometimes progressively, embarrassing not only respiration, but also the circulation, by a tension pneumothorax kinking the vena cava. The first aid measure necessary here (and in haemothorax when this produces the same effect) is decompression of the overfilled hemithorax by inserting a chest drain. If a chest drain is not available, a wide bore needle, such as a large intravenous cannula, inserted between the ribs into the pleural cavity, will alleviate the problem, as a temporary measure. Double fractures of several adjacent ribs can result in a segment of the chest wall moving paradoxically, so-

called 'flail chest', causing inefficient ventilation and gaseous exchange. The impact of a blow directly to the chest can damage the soft tissue of the lung without necessarily causing obvious damage to the chest wall. The effects do not become apparent until the second day after such an injury, when pulmonary function begins to deteriorate and serial chest radiographs show progressive consolidation of the lung. The state is usually irreversible and is known as the 'adult respiratory distress syndrome' (ARDS). High doses of anti-inflammatory corticosteroid drugs, such as prednisolone, given in advance of the development of the gross radiological signs, may prevent the fulminating deterioration of this type of injury.

Circulation
Circulation means both output and return of blood, which depends on adequacy of the:
Pump,
Rate,
Volume.
1. When the myocardial muscle, which is the pump wall, is weakened suddenly, which can be by either infarction, ischaemia or trauma, the circulation is reduced. Any of these can cause arrest of the heart, in which unconsciousness is accompanied by loss of the pulse. In these circumstances the easiest site to check this is at the carotid arteries in the neck. Loss of colour (particularly from mucous membranes) and progressive dilatation of the pupils of the eyes secondary to cerebral ischaemia also occur. After cardiac arrest, the circulation can be maintained temporarily by external cardiac massage, which is most effectively done with the patient supine on a firm surface such as the floor. It must be initiated without delay.
2. The commonest emergency requiring first aid is where a patient faints—a *vasovagal attack*, in which the vagus is excessively stimulated. The heart rate is thereby slowed to such a degree that cerebral oxygenation is not maintained. All that is necessary is to position the patient so that the head is the most dependent part, gravity assisting in bringing it blood. *Unless this is done promptly and maintained, patients can have a convulsion ('epileptic seizure' or 'fit'), sustain brain damage or even die.*
3. The volume of blood in the vasculature has to be maintained for circulation to continue. It can be reduced critically in fluid-losing

conditions such as haemorrhage, burns and excessive gastrointestinal losses, e.g. vomiting or diarrhoea.

When haemorrhage is external, it is usually possible to distinguish whether it is arterial or venous in origin. Arterial bleeding
requires strong, precise pressure to control it, with intermittent,
brief (for a few seconds) release to avoid damage from ischaemia
to an extremity beyond the pressure point. Venous bleeding can be
controlled by posture, with elevation of the site, and light pressure,
such as can be given by a gently applied bandage. If the pressure is
too tight, venous bleeding can be exacerbated by increasing back
pressure, as is developed by the use of a tourniquet in taking a
venous sample of blood.

A principle in the correction of hypovolaemia is that the fluid
used for replacement (usually given intravenously) is, as far as possible, identical with that which was lost. Thus, after haemorrhage
whole blood should be given; after burns, plasma; and for diarrhoea and vomiting, potassium-enriched saline. Some intravenous
fluids are classified as *colloids*, e.g. plasma and a number of syn-
thetics known as plasma expanders. These, by virtue of the size
of their particles, tend to hold water molecules in the circulation
better than do solutions of electrolytes, e.g. saline, classified as
crystalloids.

The same effect as occurs in losses from the vasculature is observed where blood is prevented from returning to the heart by
mechanical means, e.g. after injury to the chest the mediastinum
can be displaced by blood in one side of the thorax (haemothorax)
kinking the vena cava such that blood is prevented from returning to
the right atrium and ventricles for recirculation. The treatment is
as described above for tension pneumothorax (p.8).

Nervous system

The brain is susceptible to damage from inadequate oxygen supply,
even if this is only of short duration, i.e. in excess of four minutes.
Also, just like the vital structures of the mediastinum, the brain can
be damaged by compression. Head injury, either with or without a
fractured skull, can cause intracranial haemorrhage, most frequently
due to tearing of the middle meningeal artery. Any patient who has
had a head injury, particularly if there has been concussion (i.e. a
period of amnesia), should have regular recordings made of: degree
of responsiveness, pupillary response to light, pulse, blood pressure

and respiration rate. Surgical decompression, releasing the accumulating haematoma and clipping the bleeding vessel, must be performed
rapidly through a suitably sited burr hole. The physical signs of such a
problem include slowing of the pulse, reduced level of responsiveness,
perhaps progressing to coma, convulsions, neck stiffness and unequal
size of the pupils, with the dilated one being unresponsive to light.

In addition to the maintenance of adequate cerebral oxygenation by
cardiopulmonary resuscitation (p.50), in an emergency, care must be
taken to avoid damage to any part of the nervous system. This is especially important in the injured and unconscious patient. In moving
such a patient, it is *vital* that no flexion, extension or twisting of *any*
part of the spine be allowed. This means that, before transporting
such a patient, the spine should be splinted effectively in the position
the patient is found, to minimize damage to the spinal cord from
any fractures which may be present. Similar considerations apply to
movement of limbs, where the integrity of peripheral nerves must be
remembered. Paradoxically, any patients who are unable to change
their own position after stabilization of vital structures should be
moved at regular intervals so that the parts of the body bearing their
weight is varied and pressure sores thereby prevented.

Spinal decompression can be necessary when the spinal cord is
threatened. Usually, this is by a deposit of a malignancy such as a
lymphoma, myeloma or a secondary tumour from a primary site such
as the breast.

General effects of injury
A patient who might require emergency surgery, such as someone
recently injured, should *not* be given anything to drink, as this could
either cause inhalation or lead to delay in operation. Adequate hydration is nevertheless most important, since there is a definite risk
of acute tubular necrosis in patients who are hypotensive from hypovolaemia. Intravenous infusion can easily be part of first aid to the
injured and where indicated, e.g. multiple injury, can include blood
transfusion. Analgesia is essential at an early stage after severe injuries, especially burns, in patients who remain conscious. A strong
analgesic of the opiate type is required. Except in patients with head
injuries, small doses of morphine, of the order of 3–4 mg given slowly into a vein, is a convenient way of giving adequate relief without
dangerous respiratory depression. Conservation of heat from injured
and unconscious patients can not only improve well-being, but it

also reduces energy requirements and gives protection against hypothermia. Light-weight blankets, as used in space missions, are now
available in many ambulances and first aid kits.

Metabolic response to injury and anaesthesia

Injury, whether accidental or intentional, induces in the body a systemic response, the extent and duration of which is proportional to
the degree of the injury. This response, which occurs in the metabolism of the body, can be thought of in evolutionary terms as enabling
the injured organism to conserve and utilize its bodily function re-
sources at a time when its capacity to replenish these is diminished.
Thus, after injury the body uses as its source of energy its own fat and
protein, a process called *catabolism*. At the same time, it reduces its
urinary output of sodium chloride and water. This means it is to be
expected that urine output will fall in the immediate period after an
operation, usually for up to 2 days. The mechanisms by which this is
achieved are complex, involving changes in the function of the kidneys
and redistribution of body electrolytes and fluids. It is important to
realize that these effects cannot be reversed, even by such modern
techniques as intravenous infusion, and such could easily result in
fluid overload, if this *obligatory* response to trauma is disregarded.

Although fat seems the obvious substance to use as a source of
innate calories, the human body seems to be able to metabolize protein, particularly muscle mass, more readily. This leads to increased
excretion of nitrogenous waste products in the catabolic phase following injury. The intake and output of nitrogen can be measured
relatively easily, giving a quantitative expression of protein turnover
called *nitrogen balance*. After injury, nitrogen balance is said to be
negative, meaning that more nitrogen is put out than taken in. After
minor injury, of the size of an uncomplicated hernia repair, this lasts
for one day. After a partial gastrectomy, it lasts for 5 days. After
multiple injury involving fractures as well as soft tissue injuries,
negative nitrogen balance might continue for at least 10 days. Burns
have the same effect, extensive areas of skin loss being capable of
causing nitrogen losses well in excess of dietary intake and this process can continue for many weeks. Nitrogen loss after injury does not
occur in patients with impaired adrenal function, e.g. either those
with Addison's disease (p.147) or those who have undergone adrenalectomy.

The electrolyte potassium tends to be lost and gained in parallel with nitrogen balancing and so has to be thought of separately from

sodium. Potassium can be lost from the body in diarrhoea and other conditions where gastrointestinal fluids are lost excessively. Several diuretics (p.41) in common use increase the urinary excretion of potassium. These factors, taken with the tendency of the body to lose potassium after injury, mean that close monitoring, and frequently replacement of this electrolyte, is essential in post-operative patients.

Immobilization of parts or the whole of the body has different metabolic effects from those of trauma. These are chiefly loss of what might be thought of as bone electrolytes, calcium and phosphorus, with relatively little loss of nitrogen and potassium. Fractures cause comparable calcium losses to those of immobilization but, as is to be expected, also cause nitrogen and potassium loss. Increased calcium and phosphorus excretion in urine can lead to calculus formation, although for this to occur the immobilization has to be prolonged for over 7 weeks. Keeping the urine more acidic, i.e. of lower pH, would reduce the tendency to stone formation in enforced immobilization.

General anaesthesia alone, even without the making of a wound, causes a metabolic response of its own—characterized by the tendency to retain salt and water, and to metabolize innate fat and protein, i.e. to cause negative nitrogen balance. In the context of surgical practice, the effects of anaesthesia and operation are additive.

Classification of 'shock'
The word *shock* is in common use in clinical practice, although its meaning in this setting is different from its general lay use. Clinically, shock implies inadequacy of the circulatory system to supply the tissues of the body with oxygen and nutrients and to remove the products of metabolism.

A simple classification of shock distinguishes four types:
Cardiogenic
Hypovolaemic
Septic
Anaphylactic

Cardiogenic shock is circulatory failure attributable to a primary inadequacy of the heart. The causes of this include weakness of the myocardial muscle, as after its infarction (p.33), and abnormalities of rhythm, such as an uncontrolled ventricular rate caused by atrial fibrillation (p.45).

Hypovolaemic shock is the result of loss of circulating fluid from the vascular compartment, such as follows a haemorrhage or burns (p.23).

Septic shock, as the name implies, has an infective cause. Usually, there are micro-organisms within the blood stream, but occasionally the same picture can result from toxins these organisms produce in the circulation. The clinical picture is similar to that in cardiogenic and hypovolaemic shock, in that the patient becomes pale, sweaty, feels faint and may become unconscious. The pulse is fast but weak (often referred to as 'thready'). In septic shock, fever is usually present. The remarkable feature of this type of shock is that the physical signs described are usually rapidly reversible by the intravenous infusion of a modest volume of crystalloid, e.g. 0.9% (physiological) saline. Blood for culture must be taken immediately and the source of sepsis located and dealt with, otherwise a further episode of shock, which will be more difficult to reverse, will follow the initial resuscitation.

Anaphylactic shock (p.105) is the dramatic, intense expression by the body of *hypersensitivity* to some foreign material, usually a drug, which has been administered parenterally. The possibility of ana-phylactic reaction should be considered whenever a drug is given by injection, especially when the intravenous route is used. Fortunate-ly, it is relatively rare, but all dentists should be prepared to treat it. People who have eczema or asthma, i.e. *atopic* subjects, are particu-larly susceptible. The signs can be subdivided into mild (anaphylactic hypersensitivity) and severe (generalized anaphylaxis). Mild manifes-tations are runny nose, itch, skin rash, abdominal pain, diarrhoea and vomiting. In the severe form, the picture of shock is seen with sudden fall in blood pressure (due to vasodilatation) and mucosal and skin oedema, together with wheeze from bronchospasm. Reduced cardiac output can cause secondary myocardial insufficiency, with arrhyth-mias. Treatment requires immediate *intramuscular* adrenaline, i.e. 1 ml of 1 in 1000 (which is 1 mg/ml). This causes constriction of the peripheral blood vessels, may prevent further release of chemicals which cause the reaction, and possibly acts as a bronchodilator. This injection can be repeated at intervals of 15 minutes. Second line treat-ment is to give, immediately after the intramuscular adrenaline, by slow *intravenous* injection, an antihistamine, e.g. chlorpheniramine, 10–20 mg, to improve the oedema and skin features.

Intravenous corticosteroids, e.g. hydrocortisone hemisuccinate 200 mg, given early on, may help to prevent deterioration.

If circulatory collapse persists, it will be necessary to give intravenous fluids to expand the plasma volume. Bronchospasm may be so severe as to require intravenous aminophylline 250 mg over 10 minutes or a nebulized β_2-adrenoceptor agonist like salbutamol.

If respiratory obstruction occurs because of laryngeal oedema, emergency tracheostomy may be necessary(p.288) since it may be impossible to insert an endotracheal tube.

3 Injury: fractures, wound healing, plastic surgery and blood transfusion

Fractures

For practical purposes, fractures are classified as:

Simple or *closed* are terms used to mean that there is no communication between the break in the bone and the exterior, i.e. no wound communicating between the skin and the fracture.

Compound or *open*, when there is a breach in the integument through which dirt or organisms can pass directly to the broken bone.

Comminuted means the bone is broken in more than one place. This can increase instability and make complete reduction of the fracture and correction of deformity more difficult to achieve.

Impacted implies that the fragments resulting from fracture are driven together. This may mean that there is no instability but it can cause deformity, and, especially in long bones, shortening.

Certain types of fractures have their own distinctive features and problems:

Greenstick fractures are ones where the bone bends but without actual fragmentation or separation. This type is usually seen in the long bones of children.

Pathological fractures occur at the site of a disease process in the bone—most commonly tumour. Here the fracture may result in the course of normal usage with minimal injury or force having occurred.

Most fractures involve some loss of blood. This is often concealed. The amount of hidden haemorrhage is proportional to the size of the

16

bone broken. A working guide for calculating roughly such losses in adults is:

humerus or tibia	500 ml
shaft of femur	1000 ml
pelvis (depending on site and extent)	1000–2000 ml

Most fractures heal by the initial formation of *callus* which is a modified form of granulation tissue. Where there is incomplete immobilization of a fracture, e.g. in a rib, callus gives rise to cartilage. Usually it becomes bone which, by a process of remodelling, is ultimately indistinguishable from the original.

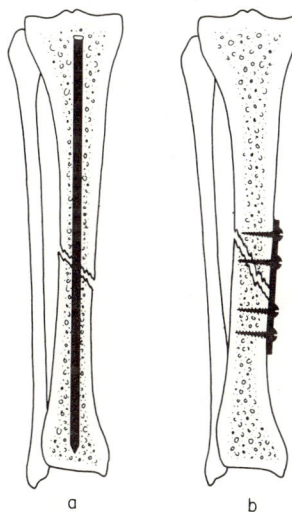

Fig. 1 Internal fixation of fractures. (a) Intramedullary nail, (b) plate and screws.

Healing of fractures can be *delayed*, usually by the persistence of haematoma. *Non-union* results when the fractured fragments are separated by soft tissue such as fascia or muscle. This can be utilized surgically, e.g. in creating a new temporomandibular joint. Delayed union and non-union can be treated by operative intervention, including *internal fixation* (Fig. 1) where inert metal nails, rods or plates are used to approximate and splint the broken fragments. *Avascular necrosis* is a particularly serious complication of a fracture, usually arising where the fracture has resulted in a vital part of a bone, e.g. the head of the femur, becoming separated from its main blood supply. It crumbles, and when stressed, by either weight bearing or the pull of surrounding muscles, it collapses, which eventually leads to intractable osteoarthritis, with attendant loss of function and pain. This diagnosis can be made from radiographs taken between one and three months after injury. The affected fragment shows by virtue of having a relatively greater density than the surrounding damaged bone at this time after the fracture, since without a blood supply, it cannot become osteoporotic. Once recognized, early operative removal, and reconstruction of the joint, either by arthroplasty or prosthesis, is important, otherwise the neighbouring joint surfaces will be irrevocably destroyed.

Pseudarthrosis is the development of a false joint at the site of a fracture, where there has been excessive movement and the cells in the callus differentiate into a synovial membrane. *Pseudofractures* are the radiological appearances of a fracture which can occur in osteomalacia (p.151) but where there is no actual breach of the bone.

Osteomyelitis means infection of the bone. It is a serious condition because it is difficult to eradicate the organisms which are of the pus-forming *pyogenic* type, usually *Staphylococcus aureus*. Most commonly, these gain entry at the time of injury, when a fracture is of the compound type, i.e. with the bone exposed to the atmosphere. Occasionally, however, blood-borne organisms can cause osteomyelitis. Infection may result in loss of blood supply to the bone, part of which may die (as in avascular necrosis) and form a contaminating particle called a *sequestrum*. Such within a fracture site results in a chronic discharge of pus (*sinus*), delayed healing and causes deformity.

   The essential aspect of treatment of osteomyelitis is adequate drainage, any potential pockets where pus might pool being opened by incision and removal of the surrounding tissue. The wound is left open, although the affected part should be immobilized. Rest and antibiotic therapy complete the management of the acute phase. If osteomyelitis becomes chronic, multiple cavities and sequestra form. More radical surgery is necessary to eliminate this, consisting of removal of all the sequestra, deroofing (*saucerization*) of the large

cavities in the bone, and obliteration of the resulting spaces by means of muscle flaps or even bone grafts.

Facial fractures

By definition, injuries to the face are head injuries. The recognition of fractures of the frontal, ethmoidal and sphenoidal air sinuses is vital, so that meningitis can be prevented by giving prophylactic antibiotics. Sometimes leakage of cerebrospinal fluid down the nose (*rhinorrhoea*) is the only sign of such fractures, but one which must be looked for carefully.

In managing facio-maxillary injuries, maintenance of an unobstructed airway is the first priority. To achieve this a tracheostomy may be indicated in:
1. Extensive facial injuries,
2. The combination of persisting reduced level of consciousness with a fractured mandible, particularly where fracture is bilateral,
3. Co-existent bronchitis (p.61) or bronchiectasis (p.60) causing copious bronchial secretions.

General anaesthesia is best avoided in the early period following head injury.

Traumatic cranial nerve injuries of dental importance

Trigeminal (5th) nerve

The infra-orbital branch of the trigeminal nerve may be damaged in association with fractures of the zygoma or the maxilla. Initially these fractures may be obscured by soft tissue swelling, but the nerve injury produces anaesthesia of the upper lip. Fractures of the middle cranial fossa may damage the more proximal parts of the nerve or the trigeminal ganglion and some permanent alteration in facial sensation usually results.

Facial (7th) nerve

Facial paralysis may occur immediately following a head injury due to interruption of the lower motor neurone fibres, when the bony canal, through which the nerve leaves the skull, is fractured. Facial paralysis of delayed onset has a better chance of recovery than the

immediate type, as in this case the cause is thought to be oedema of the nerve or bleeding within its bony canal. Injury to the nerve within the facial canal may also result in loss of taste over the anterior two-thirds of the tongue.

Patients with multiple injuries

Frequently, patients with facio-maxillary problems have multiple injuries. As a member of the team dealing with such a patient, the concept of the whole person must be kept in mind. It is useful for one member of the team managing such a patient to be in overall charge and responsible for the coordination and implementation of the management contributed by the various specialties. Exactly which specialist this is depends upon the individual circumstances and on the particular injuries present, e.g. there are times when it is most appropriately an anaesthetist, others when it is an orthopaedic surgeon or a neurosurgeon, but the cooperation by individuals working as a'team is vital for the best interests of these patients.

The order of priorities for dealing with such a patient with multiple injuries is:

Airway,
Head and cervical spine,
Chest,
Great vessels,
Abdomen,
Face,
Limbs.

Wound healing

In addition to the eight items listed in Chapter 1 (p.6) for preventing dehiscence of surgical incisions, a number of other considerations are important about wounds in surgical practice.

Trauma frequently causes particularly bad wounds. Such wounds are never sharply incised in a skin crease under aseptic conditions. Instead, they are bruised, perhaps partly torn, irregular in depth and direction, probably with some loss of tissue, and almost certainly dirty and therefore potentially infected. In addition to the measures necessary to prevent systemic infection by *Clostridiae* (*tetani* and *welchii*), traumatic wounds require *debridement*, by which is meant the

meticulous removal of all foreign material such as dirt and glass, all tissue which has been rendered irreversibly ischaemic, and that which has become infected if there has been any delay in presentation. When wounds are infected, and frequently following debridement after any traumatic laceration, wounds are left unsutured and instead *packed* with gauze soaked in antiseptic dilute sodium hypochlorite solution (0.5%) mixed with liquid paraffin to lubricate the pack and delay its drying out, thus making its later removal easier.

After this, either of two courses can be followed, depending on a number of factors. The wound can either be closed at 48 or 72 hours after debridement (*delayed primary closure*) or it can be left open (albeit packed regularly) to heal by what is called *secondary intention*. An essential prerequisite for delayed primary closure is that there is no significant loss of tissue, particularly epithelium, and that this can be accurately approximated without causing ischaemia and suture tension. Such a wound heals quickly and only a little more slowly than one closed by *primary closure*, if all other factors are equal. The healing of a wound by secondary intention is a slower, although similar reparative process. The tissue defect is initially filled with blood which clots: macrophages migrate into the clot and *granulation tissue* forms. Granulation tissue is very vascular and rich in fibroblasts, but it does not have sensory nerve fibres. The wound then contracts, its entire surface consisting of granulation tissue which is easily traumatized, but not now easily infected. The granulation tissue slowly becomes covered by epithelium which migrates to its surface, both from its edges and from the bases of any hair follicles and sweat glands which survive in the tissue deep to the wound. In the skin, the scar is formed which is initially pink and often concave, but eventually it becomes whiter and flatter.

Several factors can delay the wound healing. An inadequate blood supply can have either a local cause, e.g. diabetic arteriopathy, or a systemic cause, e.g. heart failure. Weight bearing areas and skin which has been irradiated heal poorly. Old age may itself predispose to slow healing, although this may merely be an expression of nutritional and circulatory factors. As with fractures, excessive movement of skin wounds delays healing. Irritating factors, such as foreign bodies, infection and slough, delay healing, as does failure of major organs such as the kidney and liver. Diabetics usually show poor wound healing.

Prominent *hypertrophic* scars consisting of fibrous *keloid* often develop when incisions are made in the neck or over the sternum.

Younger patients, especially girls and negroes, are specially prone to this complication, which is also common after burns.

Certain types of wounds encountered in surgery may be defined as follows:

Ulcer: discontinuity of an epithelial surface,

Fissure: a slit-like ulcer,

Sinus: a *blind* track, lined with granulation tissue, opening from an epithelial surface into surrounding tissues,

Fistula: an abnormal communication between the lumen of a viscus and an external or internal surface (including the lumen of another viscus, e.g. an oro-antral or gastro-colic fistula).

The causes of persistence of a sinus or fistula include:

1. Foreign body or dead tissue,
2. Inadequate drainage,
3. Chronic exposure to inflammation-inducing agents,
4. Obstruction of the lumen distal to the fistula,
5. Wall becoming lined with epithelium,
6. Surrounding dense fibrous tissue preventing closure,
7. Specific organisms, e.g. tubercle bacillus or actinomycetes,
8. Presence of malignant disease.

Wound infection

The development of a wound infection can be marked by signs both local and general. Local signs are *redness* (*erythema*), *hotness*, *swelling*, *pain* and *loss of function* of the affected part. Generally, the patient may become *pyrexial*, with a fast pulse (*tachycardia*), and even *toxic* (flushed or sweaty) and have an elevated white cell count (*leucocytosis*). Treatment can be as simple as removing just one suture so that accumulating pus can drain freely, through systemic antibacterial therapy, to the need to take down the entire wound to obtain adequate drainage. This latter course applies particularly if any foreign body is present in the wound, such as a prosthesis.

The virulence of the infecting organisms as well as their sensitivity to antibacterial agents influences the management, e.g. if *Clostridium welchii*, which causes gas gangrene, infects a wound, not only does this have to be taken down, but also widely excised and left open to heal by secondary intention.

Methods of reducing the risks of wound infections and surgical sepsis in general are outlined in Chapter 1 (p.4). Despite these, sometimes endogenous organisms can infect wounds which are ap-

of nines (Fig. 2) provides a rough guide to the percentage of the body surface involved. This may not always be easy to assess at the time of the initial burning injury, but its calculation may have to await the natural course of events before this declares itself by the extent and character of the loss of tissue and scars which form.

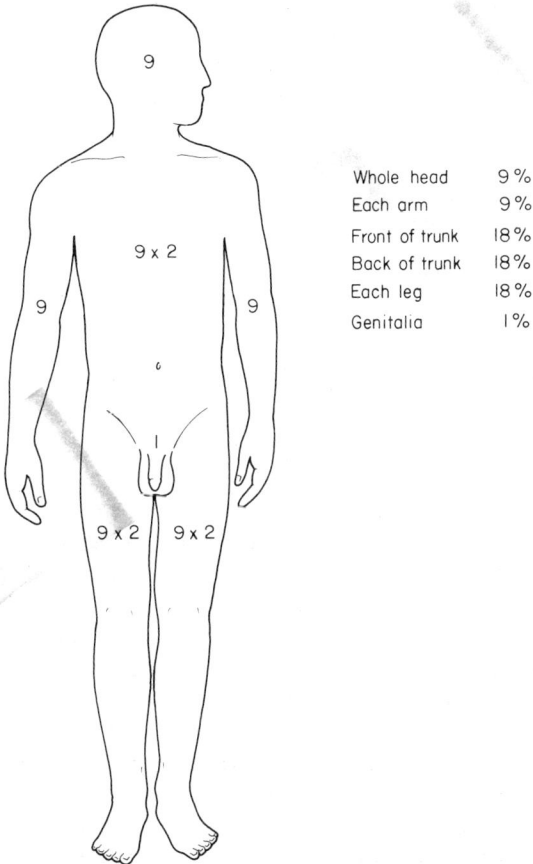

Whole head	9%
Each arm	9%
Front of trunk	18%
Back of trunk	18%
Each leg	18%
Genitalia	1%

Fig. 2 'Rule of nines' formula for estimating proportion of surface area burned in an adult. Different formulae apply for children.

Blood transfusion

Blood transfusion is essential to treat active bleeding with threatening haemorrhagic shock, by increasing both the red cell mass and parently sterile when made, the infective organisms usually being from the skin (*Staphylococcus aureus*) or gut (*E. coli*).

Plastic and reconstructive surgery

Correction of the functional aftermath of accidents to the limbs and trunk is in the realm of orthopaedic and general surgeons, but much restoration of appearance and structure is done by so-called plastic surgeons with whom oral surgeons have a specially close liaison. The highly specialized areas of their respective interests such as reconstruction of the face cannot be included in this short general textbook. Nevertheless, a few basic principles of plastic surgery can usefully be applied in other branches of surgery, including dentistry.

Modification of wounds, either for cosmetic improvement or to restore normal function, is invaluable. The simplest example is *Z-plasty*, by means of which (1) skin can be removed more widely, without fear of dehiscence, and (2) the direction and shape of scars can be changed: a vertical scar can, for example, be made horizontal. This can also enable greater margins of excision than simple bielliptical incisions would allow. Another example is the *advancement of flaps*, e.g. bringing a triangle of skin into a linear defect and so reducing tension. Beyond these simple manoeuvres, many much more complex types of flaps, such as *transposition*, are available both for skin cover and for restoration of altered anatomy.

The other important task of the plastic surgeon is in the management of burns. The systemic aspects have already been covered (p.10). As long as the burns are only of *partial thickness*, i.e. some epithelial remnants are left in hair follicles and sweat glands beneath the burned skin (in other words, the full thickness of the skin has not been destroyed), spontaneous recovery can be expected. The interval before this happens can be filled by temporary grafting with material such as porcine (pig) skin.

Full thickness of skin loss, i.e. extending below the dermis, can never recover spontaneously. It requires, once the patient's general condition is stable, excision of the destroyed skin and either replacement of this by split skin grafts or by means of musculocutaneous flaps, whereby an island of skin attached to its underlying muscle, each with its own arterial supply, is used to fill the defect.

The proportion of the whole body surface that is burned is important both for the immediate assessment and calculation of the intravenous infusion required, and for the prognosis. The *rule* cavities in the bone, and obliteration of the resulting spaces by means of muscle flaps or even bone grafts.

Facial fractures

By definition, injuries to the face are head injuries. The recognition of fractures of the frontal, ethmoidal and sphenoidal air sinuses is vital, so that meningitis can be prevented by giving prophylactic antibiotics. Sometimes leakage of cerebrospinal fluid down the nose (*rhinorrhoea*) is the only sign of such fractures, but one which must be looked for carefully.

In managing facio-maxillary injuries, maintenance of an unobstructed airway is the first priority. To achieve this a tracheostomy may be indicated in:
1. Extensive facial injuries,
2. The combination of persisting reduced level of consciousness with a fractured mandible, particularly where fracture is bilateral,
3. Co-existent bronchitis (p.61) or bronchiectasis (p.60) causing copious bronchial secretions.

General anaesthesia is best avoided in the early period following head injury.

Traumatic cranial nerve injuries of dental importance

Trigeminal (5th) nerve

The infra-orbital branch of the trigeminal nerve may be damaged in association with fractures of the zygoma or the maxilla. Initially these fractures may be obscured by soft tissue swelling, but the nerve injury produces anaesthesia of the upper lip. Fractures of the middle cranial fossa may damage the more proximal parts of the nerve or the trigeminal ganglion and some permanent alteration in facial sensation usually results.

Facial (7th) nerve

Facial paralysis may occur immediately following a head injury due to interruption of the lower motor neurone fibres, when the bony canal, through which the nerve leaves the skull, is fractured. Facial paralysis of delayed onset has a better chance of recovery than the immediate type, as in this case the cause is thought to be oedema of the nerve or bleeding within its bony canal. Injury to the nerve within the facial canal may also result in loss of taste over the anterior two-thirds of the tongue.

Patients with multiple injuries

Frequently, patients with facio-maxillary problems have multiple injuries. As a member of the team dealing with such a patient, the concept of the whole person must be kept in mind. It is useful for one member of the team managing such a patient to be in overall charge and responsible for the coordination and implementation of the management contributed by the various specialties. Exactly which specialist this is depends upon the individual circumstances and on the particular injuries present, e.g. there are times when it is most appropriately an anaesthetist, others when it is an orthopaedic surgeon or a neurosurgeon, but the cooperation by individuals working as a team is vital for the best interests of these patients.

The order of priorities for dealing with such a patient with multiple injuries is:

Airway,
Head and cervical spine,
Chest,
Great vessels,
Abdomen,
Face,
Limbs.

Wound healing

In addition to the eight items listed in Chapter 1 (p.6) for preventing dehiscence of surgical incisions, a number of other considerations are important about wounds in surgical practice.

Trauma frequently causes particularly bad wounds. Such wounds are never sharply incised in a skin crease under aseptic conditions. Instead, they are bruised, perhaps partly torn, irregular in depth and direction, probably with some loss of tissue, and almost certainly dirty and therefore potentially infected. In addition to the measures necessary to prevent systemic infection by *Clostridiae* (*tetani* and *welchii*), traumatic wounds require *debridement*, by which is meant the plasma volume and in certain severe anaemias to increase red cell mass and improve oxygen carrying capacity.

1. It is essential in the management of major traumatic and obstetric haemorrhage.
2. To enable the performance of major surgery, e.g. cardiac and vascular, major orthopaedic, and organ transplantation.
3. As part of the surgical and medical management of chronic blood loss.
4. To assist the survival of grossly anaemic infants by the use of fresh blood for intrauterine exchange and neonatal transfusion.
5. To provide long-term life-saving treatment in severe hereditary anaemias, such as severe forms of thalassaemia, and sickle cell disease (p.296).
6. To provide support through periods of bone marrow depression in chronic disease, malignancy and intensive chemotherapy.

Blood transfusion is valuable and often life-saving. It is also potentially hazardous, and whenever it is proposed, the indications and their alternatives should be carefully considered, e.g. saline or plasma solution may be sufficient to restore small blood losses and haematinics sufficient to restore haemoglobin, e.g. ferrous sulphate tablets in severe iron deficiency anaemia. Although hazards such as transmission of bacterial disease, febrile and allergic reactions and immune sensitization do occur, the most dangerous and potentially lethal are haemolytic transfusion reactions. These may be due to incorrect identification of blood sample or patient, leading to the transfusion of incompatible blood, and incorrect storage or usage, leading to the transfusion of lysed or infected blood.

It cannot be too highly emphasized that meticulous care is essential in the correct identification of the patient requiring transfusion; full and correct labelling at the bedside of the sample taken, careful recording and checking thoughout laboratory preparation, and again when the blood is about to be administered to the patient. Positive patient identification by the use of wristband label is almost universally used, and it should be referred to whenever samples are taken or treatment is about to be given to the patient.

To keep pace with advances in treatment, the concept of blood component therapy has developed. This refers to the transfusion, selectively, of the blood fractions which the patient needs, e.g. clotting factor concentrates in haemophilia, platelets for bleeding due to thrombocytopenia, without overloading the patient's circulation by also giving those parts of the blood which he can make for himself.

In Britain the provision of blood and blood products is the respon-
sibility of the Blood Transfusion Service. Its Regional Transfusion
Centres recruit panels of blood donors, collect the donations, and
carry out extensive laboratory testing to ascertain the correct ABO
and Rhesus group of each donation. Tests for *hepatitis B surface
antigen*, *syphilis* and *acquired immune deficiency syndrome* (AIDS)
are carried out. Other conditions are excluded on donor history. The
centres prepare and distribute for clinical use whole blood, red cell
concentrates, platelet concentrates, cryoprecipitate, fresh frozen
plasma, leucocyte concentrates and special red cell preparations,
such as frozen, washed and leucocyte-poor blood. They also separate
plasma to send to the two UK plasma fractioning centres for further
processing. From fresh frozen plasma come concentrates of Factor
VIII and Factor IX for the treatment of haemophilia; from expired
plasma, plasma protein solution, i.e. 4.5% albumin in saline; also 20%
albumin and normal immunoglobulin and several minor fractions.
From immune plasma, specific immunoglobulins are derived—most
importantly, anti-D immunoglobulin (for the prevention of Rhesus
sensitization), anti-tetanus immunoglobulin, anti-rabies immunoglobulin and, mainly for the treatment of immunosuppressed patients,
measles, rubella and zoster immunoglobulin.

4 Cardiovascular diseases

The basic cardiac anatomy is illustrated in Fig. 3. Venous blood enters the right atrium and progresses through the right ventricle to the pulmonary circulation where it receives oxygen and gives up carbon dioxide. It then enters the left atrium and left ventricle, from where it is pumped round the body. The left ventricle is the main pumping chamber of the heart, and disease affecting this chamber has the most serious effect.

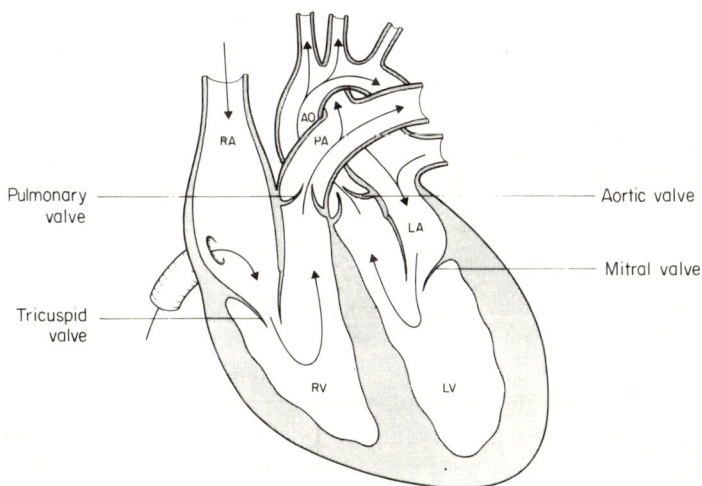

Fig. 3 Basic anatomy of the heart. RA, right atrium; RV, right ventricle; LA, left atrium; LV, left ventricle; PA, pulmonary artery; AO, aorta.

Cardiac symptoms
Although the heart may be affected by many diseases, there are a limited number of symptoms which can result.

Chest pain
This is a common symptom of cardiac disease. The patient with
angina (caused by myocardial ischaemia due to coronary atheroma)
complains of a tight, gripping pain situated behind the sternum,
possibly radiating to other areas (shoulders, arms, neck, jaw and
back). This pain is usually worst during exertion (especially in cold
weather or after heavy meals) or with emotional upset, and is relieved
by rest. The pain of a myocardial infarction, although similar in
character, is more severe, more prolonged (usually over 30 minutes)
and may be associated with sweating, nausea and dyspnoea.

Pericarditis causes central chest pain, often sharp in character
and usually worse on respiration. It may be eased by sitting up and
leaning forward. It often radiates to the neck and left shoulder, and
may therefore mimic the pain of coronary heart disease.

Other causes of chest pain include dissection of the aorta (sudden
onset of severe 'tearing' chest pain radiating to the back, caused by the
tracking of blood into the aortic wall), pleuritic pain (sharp, unilateral and worse on inspiration), musculoskeletal pain (altered by
posture, with local tenderness), and oesophageal spasm (due to
gastro-oesophageal reflux and often very like the pain of angina).

Breathlessness (dyspnoea)
This is a common symptom of pulmonary congestion due to cardiac
failure. It may occur only on exertion but in more severe heart disease occurs at rest. Orthopnoea is a 'choking' feeling which occurs
when supine, and at a later stage, the patient may experience *paroxysmal nocturnal dyspnoea* (waking with acute dyspnoea due to
increased venous return from the legs, and eased by standing up).

The other main cause of dyspnoea is pulmonary disease—features
associated with this cause might include a history of smoking or
exposure to dusts, chronic cough with sputum, and wheeze. Chest
X-ray and tests of respiratory function are often helpful in distin-
guishing this from cardiac disease.

Fatigue
This non-specific symptom occurs in cardiac failure, as well as in
many other conditions.

Palpitations
An unusual awareness of the heart beat which usually indicates an
abnormality of the cardiac rhythm, but can occur in normal subjects.

The patient may be able to tell whether the heart is beating regularly or irregularly, fast or slow, which can help with diagnosis.

Ankle swelling (oedema)
This may be due to heart failure, although there are many other causes (including kidney and liver disease).

Syncope (loss of consciousness)
There are many causes, but the cardiac ones are important, and include arrhythmias (tachycardias or, more commonly, bradycardias), and aortic stenosis.

Most episodes are, however, simple vasovagal or fainting attacks, which are characterized by a slow pulse and rapid resumption of consciousness on lying supine. These episodes may be stimulated by fear, pain, lack of food, prolonged standing or heat (p.178).

Cardiac signs
General features of the patient with cardiac disease include cyanosis (blue discolouration of the lips and tongue due to decreased oxygenation of the blood), rapid breathing and sweating.

Pulse
For convenience the radial pulse is usually examined, although the larger arteries, e.g. carotid, give a better appreciation of the pulse and are useful in emergencies, when the pulse may be weak. Features to be noted include:
1. *Rate.* The normal pulse rate lies between 60 and 100 beats/min. Faster rates (tachycardia) are usually related to emotional upset or exertion, but also occur in the presence of fever or cardiac failure, or may be due to a cardiac arrhythmia. Bradycardia (less than 60 per minute) is normal in fit, young people, but may, especially in the older subject, be due to heart block or the use of drugs, e.g. beta-blockers, digoxin.
2. *Rhythm.* This is usually regular, although children and young adults usually have sinus arrhythmia, a phasic increase and decrease in the pulse rate, varying with respiration (*see* Arrhythmias, p.42).

Blood pressure
The ability to measure blood pressure accurately is important, not only because high blood pressure carries the risk of a number of serious disorders, such as stroke, heart failure and myocardial infarction, as

well as renal and retinal damage, but also because severe cardiac disease can lead to a fall in blood pressure (hypotension). Mercury sphygmomanometers are the most reliable type, but even these need annual checking. Aneroid sphygmomanometers are less reliable, but may be more convenient. The cuff contains an inflatable bladder which should encircle the arm and be centred over the brachial artery. Problems with measurement may occur in obese subjects, and children require smaller cuffs.

The subject should be relaxed, with the arm being supported level with the heart. A stethoscope is placed over the brachial artery and the cuff inflated to greater than the expected systolic pressure, then allowed to deflate slowly. The appearance of sounds (named *Korotkoff* sounds) indicates the level of systolic pressure, and their disappearance indicates the diastolic pressure. It is also possible to estimate the systolic pressure by palpation, by noting the level at which the radial pulse becomes palpable.

Jugular veins
Prominent pulsations in the neck may be due to systemic venous congestion, usually due to *congestive cardiac failure*. This is often associated with oedema (of the ankles in the ambulatory patient and of the sacral region in the bed-bound) and liver enlargement.

Murmurs
These are due to turbulent blood flow in the heart, usually due to valvular or congenital heart disease (pp.34 and 35).

Coronary heart disease
This is the commonest cause of death in the western world. The underlying cause is atheroma, a deposition of lipids with fibrous and cellular reaction in the wall of the arteries (Fig. 4).

This may manifest as ischaemia (when myocardial oxygen requirements outstrip the supply, as in exercise) or infarction, when death of myocardium occurs due to coronary artery blockage (often with an element of thrombosis occurring at the surface of the atheromatous plaque).

Atheroma which also affects other arteries, e.g. cerebral, lower limb, is predisposed by several 'risk factors'. The major ones are:
1. Hypertension
2. Cigarette smoking
3. High blood cholesterol

Other factors have less influence, but are also linked. These include physical inactivity, obesity, diabetes mellitus, diet (salt and fat intake), oral contraceptives (which may cause hypertension) and stress. There is also a genetic influence in the development of coronary heart disease. The incidence increases with age, and it is generally commoner in males, especially in the younger and middle-aged groups.

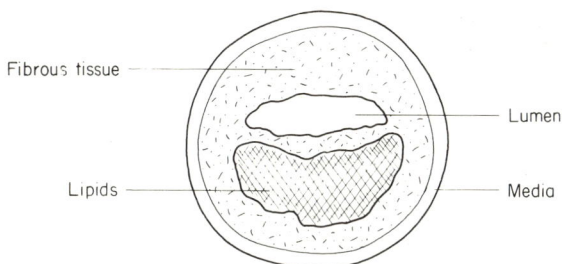

Fig. 4 Cross-section of coronary artery with atheroma.

Myocardial ischaemia
The main symptom is angina. Such patients are at risk of myocardial infarction, especially if the angina is frequent, occurs at rest (often during the night) and is responding poorly to medical treatment (unstable angina). Patients with angina may also experience cardiac arrhythmias.

Treatment
General measures:
    Stop smoking,
    Treat high blood pressure,
    Reduce weight,
    Lower high blood cholesterol (diet, drugs).

Drugs:
    1. Nitrates. Decrease cardiac workload by venodilatation and therefore decrease venous return to the heart; also dilate coronary arteries.
    Preparations include:
      Glyceryl trinitrate
        Sublingual tablet or aerosol spray used before and during pain,

Buccal, fixotropic tablets, placed between upper lip
and gum, release the nitrate slowly over a period,
Self-adhesive skin patches or ointment containing
the drug, the drug is slowly absorbed through the skin.
   Isosorbide mononitrate or dinitrate
   Oral,
   Chewable for more prolonged release of the drug.
Side effects of nitrates, due to vasodilatation, include headache,
flushing and postural hypotension, especially when angina is severe
or when patients are unusually sensitive to the effects of nitrates.
2. Beta-blockers. β–adrenoceptor blockers diminish the
tachycardia of exercise. There are many preparations with varied
pharmacological profiles. Examples are propranolol, oxprenolol,
atenolol, and metoprolol.
   Side effects include:
   Fatigue, heart failure,
   Cold extremities,
   Wheezing.
The latter two are less common with the cardioselective agents
atenolol and metoprolol.
3. *Calcium-channel blockers*
   Verapamil: decreases cardiac contractility, so may cause heart
   failure,
   Nifedipine: vasodilator, decreasing cardiac workload. Side ef-
   fects are of vasodilatation—headache, flushing, oedema.
   Diltiazem.

Note. Both beta-blockers and calcium-channel blockers are also used
in the treatment of hypertension.

Surgical treatment This consists of coronary artery bypass grafting,
using the patient's own saphenous veins. It may be required if medical
treatment fails to control angina. Following surgery, patients may be
on anticoagulants or, more commonly, anti-platelet drugs (aspirin,
dipyridamole).

Myocardial infarction
Previously called *coronary thrombosis*, this usually presents with
severe central chest pain, associated with sweating, nausea and
dyspnoea. There is a high mortality, especially in the first few hours

(more than one third die before they reach hospital). Complications include:
1. *Arrhythmias*, the major cause of death being *ventricular fibrillation*.
2. *Heart failure and shock*, both with a poor prognosis.

Most patients go to a coronary care unit for about 48 hours, mainly for monitoring and treatment of arrhythmias (which are commonest in the early period after myocardial infarction).

Treatment
Adequate analgesia, e.g. diamorphine,
Oxygen,
Bed rest for a few days.

Following myocardial infarction, patients are at increased risk of further infarction and of death due to arrhythmias. General anaesthetics should be avoided for six months if possible, because of the increased risk of cardiac arrhythmias caused by anaesthetic agents, and the risk of hypotension.

Peripheral vascular disease
When atheroma affects the leg arteries, the patient may experience painful calves on walking (intermittent claudication) due to ischaemia of the leg muscles. More severe disease may lead to pain at rest, with a risk of gangrene (tissue necrosis). Peripheral vascular disease is strongly linked with cigarette smoking.
Treatment includes:
Stopping smoking,
Control of hypertension,
Encouraging exercise,
Surgery:
by-pass grafting,
sympathectomy: decreases vasoconstriction,
Drugs (vasodilators): of little proven benefit.

Raynaud's phenomenon
This occurs when spasm of arteries in the fingers causes pain and pallor, usually in cold weather. It may occur spontaneously or be related to other conditions, including the connective tissue disorders.

Cerebrovascular disease
A *cerebrovascular accident* (CVA) can be due either to *haemorrhage* (for which hypertension is a risk factor) or *thrombosis* (either *thrombosis in situ* or arterial *embolus*) and usually occurs in vessels

affected by atheroma. The effects of a CVA depend on the part of the brain involved. The commonest type is a lesion of the middle cerebral artery affecting the motor fibres in the internal capsule, causing hemiplegia (loss of power of the arm and leg on the opposite side of the body), speech defects and variable degrees of loss of consciousness. Treatment is initially supportive, but stopping smoking, control of hypertension and perhaps anti-platelet drugs are important later. *See also* p.172.

A *subarachnoid haemorrhage* may be due to the rupture of a congenital arterial aneurysm, causing leakage of blood into the subarachnoid space. This causes severe headache, neck stiffness and loss of consciousness. Surgical treatment (clipping of the base of the aneurysm) may be possible.

Transient cerebral ischaemic attacks (TCIA) are usually due to small arterial emboli, and may be recurrent. The emboli may arise from the heart or carotid arteries (when they may come from an atheromatous plaque) and the patient experiences transient neurological abnormalities, e.g. visual upsets, transient weakness of limbs. Treatment may be medical (anti-platelet drugs) or surgical, e.g. carotid endarterectomy.

Valvular heart disease
This is usually due to *rheumatic heart disease* (following rheumatic fever in childhood) although some forms may be congenital (e.g. *bicuspid aortic valve* leading to *aortic stenosis*) or *'degenerative'* (e.g. *mitral incompetence* due to *mitral leaflet prolapse*). Valves may be narrowed (stenosed) or leaking (incompetent) or both. The diagnosis is clinical, based on typical heart murmurs. The associated murmurs reflect the timing of the abnormal flow over the valves, e.g. systolic in aortic stenosis and mitral incompetence, diastolic in aortic incompetence and mitral stenosis.

The mitral valve is the one most commonly affected by rheumatic heart disease. In either stenosis or incompetence, the patient experiences dyspnoea due to pulmonary congestion. Most valve lesions cause a gradual deterioration in symptoms with heart failure as a late consequence. Aortic stenosis, however, is much more dangerous, and may lead to sudden death, often preceded by episodes of angina and syncope.

Patients with valve disease are at risk of developing *infective endocarditis* following various procedures, including dental treatment. They therefore require prophylactic antibiotics (p.38).

Definitive treatment of heart valve lesions is by surgery, which is of two types:
1. *Reconstructive*, e.g. mitral valvotomy—splitting a stenotic valve.
2. *Valve replacement* with two main types of valve being used:
   (a) *Tissue valves*, e.g. pig valves—these valves do not generally require subsequent anticoagulation (although patients with mitral valve replacement and atrial fibrillation are usually continued on anticoagulants to prevent embolism from the dilated left atrium). The life span of these valves tends to be shorter than prosthetic (mechanical) valves.
   (b) *Prosthetic valves*, e.g. tilting disc (Björk–Shiley)—these last indefinitely but the patient requires lifelong anticoagulation. Even a few days of stopping anticoagulants without control of prothrombin time or thrombotest may lead to a thrombus occluding the valve, necessitating further surgery.
All valve replacement patients require prophylactic antibiotics before dental procedures, because of the high risk of developing endocarditis in the unprotected patient (p.38).

Congenital heart disease
Although present at birth, this may only be diagnosed in later life. Abnormalities include:
1. *Shunts*, with flow of blood through abnormal communications in the heart, usually from the left side to the right, e.g. *atrial* or *ventricular septal defect, patent ductus arteriosus*.
2. *Valve defects*, e.g. *aortic* or *pulmonary stenosis*.
3. *Complex defects*, presenting in infancy, e.g. *transposition of the great arteries*.

Problems include:
   (a) Development of pulmonary hypertension and cardiac failure,
   (b) Risk of endocarditis.
Most of these defects are now amenable to surgical correction, but this does not always remove the risk of endocarditis.

Infective endocarditis
Infection of the heart valves or endocardium with blood-borne organisms is known as endocarditis. Patients with congenital cardiac abnormalities or rheumatic heart disease are particularly at risk.

Normally, organisms entering the blood stream are rapidly destroyed but damaged endothelium offers them an environment which encourages their survival and multiplication. Most cases are caused by bacteria, although other organisms, e.g. viruses or fungi, may cause endocarditis. Common sources of bacteraemia (bacteria in the blood stream) include:

1. All dental procedures, particularly extraction,
2. Apical tooth abscesses or other dental sepsis,
3. Surgery or instrumentation of gastrointestinal or genitourinary tracts,
4. Contaminated intravenous injections, e.g. heroin addicts,
5. Cardiac surgery.

Note. Severe bacteraemia with a virulent organism may cause endocarditis on a normal valve.

Infection of a valve leads to the accumulation of platelets, fibrin, cells and bacteria to form friable masses (vegetations) which help to protect the bacteria from the body's defence mechanisms and from antibiotics. Lesions prone to be complicated by endocarditis include:

(a) Rheumatic: mitral and aortic valve disease,
(b) Congenital: ventricular septal defect, patent ductus arteriosus, bicuspid aortic valve, pulmonary stenosis, coarctation of the aorta,
(c) Degenerative: mitral leaflet prolapse,
(d) Pacemakers and intracardiac prostheses.

Acute endocarditis
This form of endocarditis is caused by virulent organisms, e.g. *Staphylococcus aureus*, *Streptococcus pyogenes* or fungi. The patient's clinical condition deteriorates rapidly, and there is a high mortality.

Subacute bacterial endocarditis (SBE)
This is an illness of insidious onset with malaise, weight loss, fever and gradual deterioration in cardiac function. There is often no obvious source of the infecting organism, which is of low-grade virulence, e.g. *viridans streptococci*, *Staph. albus* or *Strep. faecalis*. The *viridans streptococci*, which are the commonest causes of bacterial endocarditis, originate from the mouth and may be penicillin-resistant, particularly in patients who have received penicillin prophylaxis for rheumatic

fever. *Strep. faecalis* is most likely to be the cause after bowel or urinary tract interference and is notable because of its total resistance to benzyl penicillin and high degree of resistance to other antibiotics. *Staph. albus* is particularly associated with cardiac prostheses.

Physical signs include those of anaemia, splinter haemorrhages (linear haemorrhages under the finger nails, caused by emboli), finger clubbing and heart murmurs (which may change character as valve destruction progresses).

Complications include:
1. Cardiac—valve incompetence leading to cardiac failure,
2. Arterial emboli from vegetations,
3. Renal damage—emboli and immune complex-mediated nephritis.

Diagnosis
1. *Blood cultures* are most important and up to 6 sets must be taken from each suspected case of endocarditis. A positive culture is obtained in approximately 60% of patients, the usual reason for failure being prior administration of antibiotics. *It is imperative that antibiotics are not given until all blood cultures have been obtained.* Positive cultures should be aimed for in all patients because the correct choice of antibiotic therapy depends on detailed antibiotic sensitivity testing.
2. *Echocardiography*—cardiac ultrasound often demonstrates the presence of vegetations on valves.
3. *Blood count* (anaemia and raised white cell count); raised erythrocyte sedimentation rate (ESR).
4. *Immune complexes* are elevated in 75% of patients and provide a useful marker for monitoring the patient's progress during therapy.

Note. This illness must be suspected in every patient with rheumatic or congenital heart disease or an intracardiac prosthesis who develops pyrexia of unknown origin, or becomes inexplicably unwell.

Treatment
1. *Antibiotics* (*see* below).
2. *Cardiac surgery* is only required when severe valve incompetence leads to cardiac failure or when recurrent embolism occurs. Valve replacement is necessary, but in the presence of active infection,

carries a high risk of prosthetic valve endocarditis; therefore surgery should be delayed, if possible, until the infection has been cured.

Antibiotic treatment of subacute bacterial endocarditis
Treatment depends on the organism involved in the infection and its susceptibility to antibiotics. Hence the requirement for isolation of the organism wherever possible. There are a few general rules which should be observed:
1. Bactericidal drugs *must* be used for treatment. There is no place for bacteriostatic agents.
2. To obtain a powerful bactericidal activity and prevent the development of resistance two drugs in combination are often required. These must both be *bactericidal* and may be synergistic. A *bactericidal and bacteriostatic combination should never be used* because the drugs will *antagonize* each other's activity.
3. Antibiotics should be given parenterally, to ensure effective blood levels, for at least 4 weeks.
4. Therapy should continue for 6–8 weeks, and should be monitored by careful clinical assessment and serial estimation of immune complex levels.

Endocarditis due to *viridans streptococci* is often treated with a combination of benzyl penicillin and gentamicin, which are usually synergistic. If the bacterial cause of the endocarditis is not known and 'best guess' choices are being made, ampicillin in combination with gentamicin is preferable to cover the possibility of *Strep. faecalis* infections. Where *Staph. albus* is involved, cloxacillin or vancomycin is required, combined with an appropriate second antibiotic if possible. The advice of a medical microbiologist is essential in selecting the most appropriate therapy and he will be able to arrange for the most useful antibiotic sensitivity tests. Failure to achieve the right treatment has dire consequences: the mortality rate of this infection is still of the order of 20%.

Antibiotic prophylaxis in endocarditis
It follows from the above that the difficulties of treatment and the serious consequences of infective endocarditis dictate that prevention should be as effective as possible. This is a difficult area because there are few clinical trials to guide the clinician in his choice of preventive

therapy and animal studies have been criticized as being irrelevant to the human disease. Nevertheless the recommendations for prophylaxis, based on wide experience, do not differ much from country to country.

The types of patient susceptible to infective endocarditis are listed above. The procedures which put these patients at risk are:

1. Dental treatment, including all procedures which cause gingival bleeding,
2. Tonsillectomy, bronchoscopy,
3. Bowel surgery; surgery or manipulation of the genito-urinary tract; endoscopy; childbirth by vaginal delivery.

Antibiotic prophylaxis should wherever possible be with bactericidal drugs and is preferably given by parenteral routes. If given orally, the taking of the drug should be supervised.

For procedures in the mouth and respiratory tract recommendations are generally as outlined in Table 1.

Table 1. Endicarditus: antibiotic prophylaxis.

Patient type	Dose schedule
Standard requirement for patients needing cover for dental treatment	A
Requirement for use when maximal protection is desired, e.g. for patients with prosthetic valves	C
For penicillin hypersensitive patients	B or D
For those who have had a course of penicillin within the previous 2 – 3 weeks including prophylaxis for rheumatic fever	B or D

A. One vial of triple Penicillin Injection BNF (a mixture of benethamine, procaine and benzyl penicillins) by intramuscular injection 15–30 min before the procedure.

alternatively
2g amoxycillin orally under supervision 1 hour before the procedure and a further 3 doses of 500 mg taken every 6 hours.

B. Cephazolin (Kefzol) 1 g and gentamicin 1.5 mg/kg body weight by separate intramuscular injection 30 min before the procedure.
alternatively
Erythromycin 1 g orally under supervision 30 min before the procedure and a further 3 doses of 500 mg taken every 6 hours.

C. Ampicillin 2.0 g plus gentamicin 1.5 mg/kg body weight, given intramuscularly or intravenously 30 min before the procedure, followed by 1.0 g amoxycillin orally 6 hours later. Alternatively, the parenteral requirement may be repeated once 8 hours later.

D. Vancomycin 1 g by *slow* intravenous infusion 30 minutes before the procedure. No repeat dose is required.

It should be noted that whilst the above recommendations will suffice for the majority of patients, instances will arise where an individual patient cannot be fitted into any of the categories. In such a case expert advice should be sought.

Heart failure
This condition is due to an inability of the heart to pump blood adequately, leading to features of diminished tissue perfusion (cold extremities, low blood pressure, impaired renal and cerebral function) and of backward congestion (pulmonary congestion in left ventricular failure, systemic venous congestion in right ventricular failure, i.e. oedema, enlarged neck veins, liver enlargement).

Secondary effects are due to salt and water retention (due to secondary hyperaldosteronism caused by diminished renal perfusion) and increased sympathetic activity, causing tachycardia and vasoconstriction.

Causes include:
Left ventricular failure
   coronary heart disease, hypertension
   mitral or aortic valve disease
Right ventricular failure
   pulmonary hypertension, e.g. chronic obstructive airways disease.
Both right and left ventricular failure may coexist.

Treatment

Treat underlying cause if possible, e.g. valve replacement, antihypertensives. Bed rest, if severe.

Drugs

Diuretics. To diminish salt and water retention by increasing renal excretion:

1. *Thiazides*, e.g. bendrofluazide, which inhibit sodium reabsorption in the cortical diluting segment of the loop of Henle and the early proximal and distal renal tubules. Unwanted effects include potassium depletion, precipitation of gout and aggravation of diabetes mellitus.
2. *Loop diuretics*, e.g. frusemide—more powerful agents which may be used intravenously or orally. Side effects are similar to those of the thiazides.
3. *Potassium sparing agents*, e.g. spironolactone, usually used with loop diuretics. Low potassium levels in the bloodstream may predispose to cardiac arrhythmias and also potentiate the toxicity of digoxin.

Digoxin is frequently used, but its effectiveness is uncertain. It increases the force of contraction of the heart, and also slows the rate of ventricular contraction in atrial fibrillation, which is its main use. Toxic effects are common, as the effective dose is close to the toxic dose, and include anorexia, nausea, vomiting and arrhythmias (tachycardias or bradycardias). Toxicity is more likely to occur in the presence of hypokalaemia (low serum potassium) or renal failure and in those of low body weight, especially the elderly. It usually responds to temporary withdrawal of the drug.

Vasodilators which decrease the workload of the heart by dilating peripheral vessels:

1. Venodilators, e.g. nitrates,
2. Arterial dilators, e.g. hydralazine—may cause hypotension,
3. Venodilator and arterial dilator, e.g. prazosin,
4. Captopril and enalapril, angiotensin converting enzyme (ACE) inhibitors, have both a vasodilating effect and also counteract salt retention.

Embolism
Passage of material from one part of the circulation to another, with
blockage of the vessel where it lodges. In thromboembolism the material is blood clot. This can occur in either the venous or arterial
system.

Venous. The embolus lodges in a pulmonary artery (*pulmonary
embolus*) and usually arises from an area of thrombosis in the leg
veins (deep venous thrombosis, DVT), or pelvic veins. DVT is predisposed by prolonged rest (e.g. after surgery, p.5) and presents with a
tender swollen leg. However, major pulmonary embolus can occur
from the pelvic veins with no prior signs in the lower limbs. The
clinical features of pulmonary embolism depend on its size:
1. Small—pleuritic chest pain, haemoptysis.
2. Large—severe central chest pain, collapse, shock.
    Treatment is with anticoagulants. The acute pulmonary embolus or
DVT is managed with a course of intravenous *heparin*, which protec-
tively coats the damaged venous endothelium as well as acting as an
anticoagulant. Subsequently, *warfarin* is continued for a period of
about three months. Long-term anticoagulants may be required for
recurring episodes (p.88).

Arterial. The embolus lodges in a systemic artery, leading to necrosis
of the area it supplies, e.g. brain (stroke), leg (ischaemia, with pain,
pallor and absent pulses, or, later, gangrene), gut, spleen or kidney
(infarction).
    The usual source is the left side of the heart, either valvular, e.g. in
endocarditis, or from thrombosis on the wall of the heart (in
the left atrium in mitral stenosis, or left ventricle after myocardial
infarction). It occasionally arises from a large artery, e.g. carotid. The
treatment of choice is surgical removal (embolectomy) if it affects a
limb. Certain affected organs, e.g. kidney or gut, may have to be
removed. It may be possible to prevent recurrence by anticoagulation, but definitive prevention is by surgical treatment of the source,
e.g. removal of ventricular aneurysm.

Arrhythmias
The normal regular rhythm of the heart is maintained by the electrical
activity of a pacemaker situated in the right atrium, the sino-atrial
node. Each impulse causes atrial contraction as it passes through

the atrial wall to the atrioventricular node, which is situated at the junction of the atria and the ventricle. The electrical impulse then passes down specialized conducting tissue (Fig. 5) and stimulates ventricular contraction. Stimulation of the vagus nerve depresses the sino-atrial node and causes slowing of the heart.

Sinus arrhythmia
The heart rate quickens during inspiration and slows down again during expiration, probably as a result of alterations in vagal tone and the return of venous blood to the heart (Fig. 6). This is a normal physiological variant and is commonly present in children and young adults.

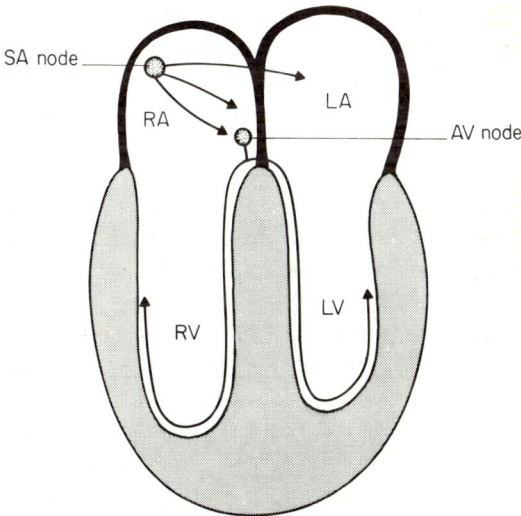

Fig. 5 Conduction system of the heart.

Extrasystoles (ectopic beats)
An extrasystole is a heart beat which originates in an abnormal focus in the heart. Extrasystoles may cause palpitations or be asymptomatic. The normal regularity of the pulse is temporarily interrupted by an

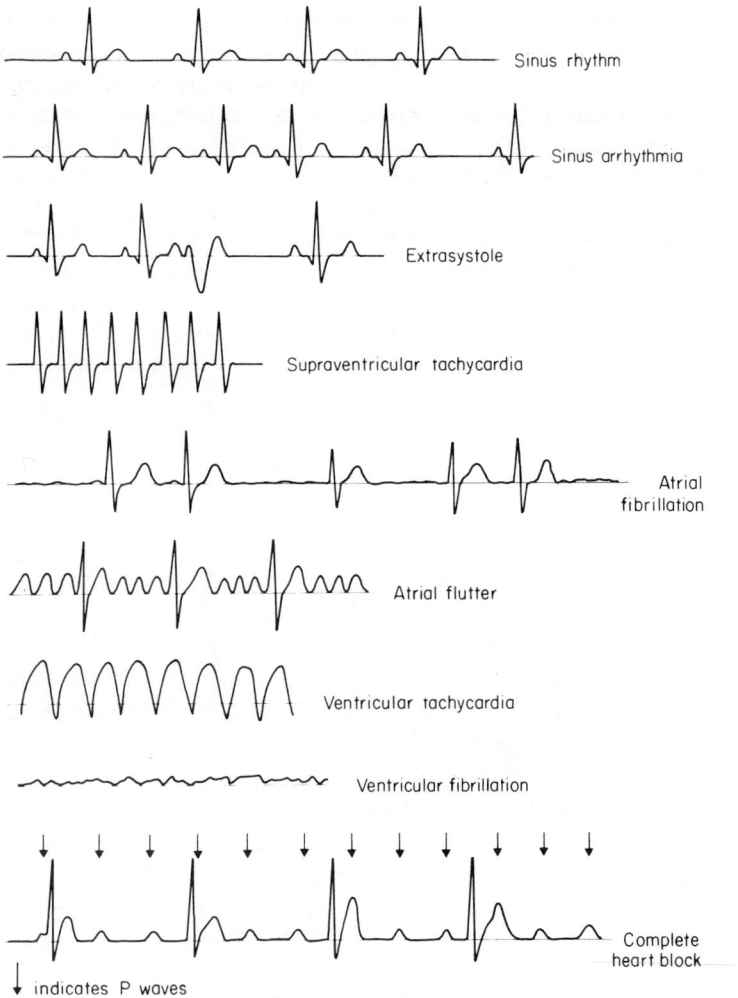

Fig. 6 Common cardiac arrhythmias.

earlier, weaker pulse, followed by a longer than normal pause. Extrasystoles may occur in a healthy person, often following excessive coffee or tobacco consumption. They commonly occur in the diseased heart, when they may be a prelude to more serious arrhythmias, usually a paroxysmal tachycardia. Extrasystoles themselves usually require no treatment.

Paroxysmal tachycardia
A fast heart rate arising from an ectopic focus in the atria or ventricles.

Atrial tachycardia (or supraventricular tachycardia, SVT)
Presents with recurrent palpitations and need not be associated with underlying heart disease. Treatment of acute attack is by vagal stimulation (slowing atrioventricular conduction), e.g. carotid sinus massage, or by drugs, e.g. verapamil, β-adrenoceptor blocker. Occasionally cardioversion may be required (application of a direct current electric shock to the chest wall, under general anaesthetic). Attacks may be prevented by these same anti-arrhythmic drugs, e.g. verapamil or β-adrenoreceptor blocker.

Ventricular tachycardia
Usually more serious than SVT, ventricular tachycardia often occurs in association with ischaemic heart disease. The patient is usually unwell, with heart failure, shock or syncope. Initial treatment is usually electrical cardioversion, followed by anti-arrhythmic drugs to prevent recurrence, e.g. lignocaine or mexiletine.

Atrial fibrillation (AF)
In this arrhythmia, atrial contraction is no longer initiated by the sino-atrial node, but takes place in a rapid, uncontrolled, chaotic manner which results in excessive and irregular stimulation of the ventricles. The pulse is totally irregular and is usually rapid in the absence of treatment. Uncontrolled AF may cause distressing palpitations and cardiac failure. Atrial emptying is impaired and the resulting stasis leads to the formation of thrombus, with the risk of systemic embolism. The most important causes of AF are mitral valve disease, ischaemic and hypertensive heart disease, and thyrotoxicosis.

Treatment
1. Digoxin to control the ventricular rate,
2. Anticoagulation to prevent emboli, especially in mitral stenosis,
3. Treat underlying cause if possible.

Atrial flutter
Closely related to AF with a rapid regular rhythm. The ventricular rate may be half or a third of the atrial rate, causing a rapid regular pulse. Treatment is with digoxin to control the ventricular rate. Cardioversion may be used in both atrial flutter and fibrillation.

Heart block

This results from interruption of normal atrioventricular conduction, due to ischaemia or fibrosis of the conducting tissue. In incomplete heart block, a ventricular beat is missed intermittently. In complete heart block, the ventricles beat independently at a very slow rate (30–49/min) or even slower at times, which may cause syncope. Such patients require a permanent pacemaker.

Hypertension

Normal arterial blood pressure tends to increase with age, but the accepted upper limit of normal for patients below the age of 65 is 140/90 mmHg. Blood pressures above normal are associated with increased morbidity and a decreased life expectancy.

Causes of hypertension

Essential hypertension. This accounts for the vast majority of cases. The cause is unknown. Salt in the diet may be important, and the primary defect may lie in the kidneys.

Secondary hypertension
1. *Renal disease*. Damage to one or both kidneys may cause hypertension, e.g. chronic renal failure (chronic glomerulonephritis or pyelonephritis), polycystic kidneys or renal artery stenosis.
2. *Endocrine causes*, e.g. Cushing's syndrome, phaeochromocytoma, Conn's syndrome (primary hyperaldosteronism).
3. *Drugs*, e.g. oral contraceptives, corticosteroids.
4. *Miscellaneous*, e.g. coarctation of the aorta, pre-eclampsia (pregnancy).

There may be no manifestation of the disease in the early stages, hypertension often being discovered at a routine medical examination. The major complications are:
(a) Cardiac—coronary heart disease, left ventricular failure,
(b) Central nervous sytem—strokes,
(c) Retinal damage, affecting vision,
(d) Chronic renal failure,
(e) Accelerated peripheral vascular disease.
Other features include headache and epistaxis.

   An attempt may be made to identify an underlying cause, especially if the hypertension occurs in the young, or is severe and difficult to control. Severe hypertension (greater than 260/140 mmHg) is known as accelerated or malignant hypertension, and carries a particularly poor prognosis, if untreated.

Treatment of hypertension

Treatment reduces the incidence of most complications (especially strokes, heart failure and renal failure) and increases life expectancy. Therapy aims to keep the diastolic pressure below 90 mmHg.

Initial management
Lose weight if obese,
Moderate salt restriction,
Decrease alcohol intake,
Stop smoking,
Stop any hypertension-producing drugs, e.g. non-steroidal anti-inflammatory drugs or the contraceptive pill.

Drug therapy

1. β-adrenoceptor blockers are usually the first choice, except where contraindicated, e.g. obstructive airways disease, peripheral vascular disease, and often in the elderly. Cardioselective preparations (atenolol, metoprolol) have fewer side effects, but all may cause cardiac failure, especially in the elderly. Many patients complain of fatigue and cold hands.
2. Thiazide diuretics, e.g. bendrofluazide, hydrochlorothiazide, are the first choice in the elderly, and are much cheaper than the β-adrenoceptor blockers. Side effects include hypokalaemia, gout, impaired glucose tolerance and impotence in the young male.
3. Vasodilators, used after a combination of the above two drugs has failed to adequately control hypertension. Examples are nifedipine, prazosin and hydralazine. They have individual side effects, but all may cause flushing and hypotension.
4. Other drugs include:
   captopril, enalapril (angiotensin converting enzyme inhibitors): these are generally well tolerated and will be used more in the future.
   methyldopa: sedation and depression may occur.

In moderate to severe hypertension, these drugs, which lower blood pressure by different mechanisms, are often used in combination, as side effects are less troublesome at lower doses, and their effects on blood pressure are at least additive.

Hypertension during pregnancy
Because of the hyperdynamic circulation in pregnancy, the Korotkoff
sounds often persist to zero pressure. It is therefore customary to
measure Phase IV (muffling) diastolic pressure. Blood pressure falls
during the first 3 months of pregnancy, is at its lowest between 16
and 20 weeks of gestation, then rises progressively until term. These
changes affect the diastolic pressure more than they do systolic
pressure.
   Blood pressure readings taken during pregnancy are dependent on
posture. Systolic pressure tends to rise in the supine position, whilst
sometimes there is a marked drop in blood pressure in this position
because of compression of the inferior vena cava by the uterus.

General anaesthesia and surgery in patients with heart disease
Most general anaesthetics depress cardiac contractility and may
therefore be harmful in patients with impaired cardiac function.
Alterations in cardiac rhythm are common during operation, and
monitoring of the electrocardiogram is desirable, especially in patients with coronary heart disease. In recent years the practice has
been extended to cover all operations under general anaesthesia.
   Some specific cardiovascular disorders which have relevance to
surgery are as follows:

Ischaemic heart disease
Elective surgery (and general anaesthetics) should be avoided for six
months after a myocardial infarction, due to the increased risk of
cardiac arrhythmias, reinfarction and death. Patients with poorly
controlled or unstable angina (pain at rest) should not have a general
anaesthetic or surgery until their angina has been treated successfully.

Hypertension
Patients with hypertension are subject to wide swings in BP during
surgery and some agents, e.g. halothane, are particularly likely to
induce dangerous hypotension. Anti-hypertensive drugs should not
be discontinued pre-operatively, and patients with severe hypertension should have this controlled before their operation.

Valvular disease
Prophylactic antibiotics are required (p.38). Anticoagulants can be discontinued for two days before and after operation in most cases. However, prosthetic (mechanical) valves are prone to thrombosis, and careful control of anticoagulant withdrawal is necessary, e.g. keeping 'thrombotest' activity between 5 and 15% (p.86).

Heart failure
This should be properly controlled before surgery, as it is associated with increased mortality.

Loss of consciousness in the dental chair
The most common cause is simple *vasovagal syncope*. Other causes, however, such as *cardiac arrest*, must be excluded. The following procedures should be adopted:
1. Ensure that the patient's airway is clear,
2. Place the patient in a horizontal position (failure to do this in a simple vasovagal attack may result in the patient having an epileptiform convulsion because of cerebral anoxia),
3. Check that a radial or carotid pulse is palpable. If no pulse can be felt, proceed as for cardiac arrest.

   Recovery from a vasovagal episode will be rapid once the patient has assumed the horizontal position.

Cardiac arrest
Cessation of effective cerebral circulation because of uncoordinated ventricular contraction (*ventricular fibrillation*) or *ventricular standstill* (*asystole*). Cardiac arrest is characterized by sudden collapse, loss of consciousness and absent pulses. The pupils start to dilate within 30–40 seconds and the patient may have a convulsion. Some of the important causes include:
1. Acute myocardial infarction,
2. Underventilation during general anaesthetic,
3. Airway obstruction,
4. Vagal reflexes initiated by tracheal stimulation, e.g. intubation or inhaled vomitus, especially in patients with ischaemic heart disease,
5. Drugs, particularly anaesthetics,
6. Electrocution.

Treatment

(a) Confirm the diagnosis by noting absent carotid pulses. This will distinguish cardiac arrest from the more common vasovagal attack.

(b) Strike the front of the chest once with the closed fist: this may restart the heart.

(c) If this fails, lie the patient flat.

(d) *External cardiac massage.* Firmly depress the lower half of the sternum $1^{1}/_{2}$–2 inches with the heels of the hands about 70 times per minute—this maintains the cardiac output by compressing the heart between the sternum and the vertebral column. A pulse should be palpable over a major artery and the pupil size should return to normal if an effective circulation is being maintained.

(e) *Artificial ventilation.* Clear the airway (including suction of vomitus), extend the neck, and pull the jaw forward. Mouth-to-mouth resuscitation should be commenced at a rate of 20 per minute, with one hand closing the patient's nostrils. A pharyngeal airway should be inserted if available. The chest must be seen to expand and the patient's colour should become pink.

These measures can maintain the patient for up to one hour while he or she is transferred to hospital.

5   Respiratory tract disorders

Anatomy and physiology
The respiratory tract can be arbitrarily divided into two distinct anatomical parts:

Upper respiratory tract which comprises the nose, paranasal air sinuses, pharynx and larynx. The principal function is to warm, humidify and conduct the inspired air to the lower respiratory tract. In addition it has important defence functions which include the actions of the hairs in the anterior part of the nose and the turbinates which cause turbulence in the air flow, both of which precipitate particulate matter from the air. Also the sneeze, cough and gag reflexes which prevent inhalation of noxious material. The pharynx is also rich in lymphatic tissue which has an immunological function.

Lower respiratory tract comprises:
1. *Conducting airways*, beginning at the trachea which divides into the two main bronchi at the carina. These divide and branch, decreasing in size as they do so, to produce the segmental bronchi, the bronchioles and eventually the terminal bronchioles. The bronchial tree is lined with a single layer of ciliated cells rich in mucous glands. On the tips of the cilia there is a thin layer of watery mucus on to which particles and irritants settle from the inspired air. The beating of the cilia moves the mucus up the bronchial tree to the larynx from where it is constantly being swallowed, thus keeping the lower airway clean and healthy. The mucus also has some bactericidal and immunological properties.
2. *Alveoli*, which are air spaces 0.25 mm in diameter, arise from the respiratory bronchioles which are branches of the terminal bronchioles. The alveoli are lined with a single layer of flattened epithelium and adjacent alveoli are separated by their respective lining epithelium and a rich capillary network. The anatomical arrangement therefore provides an enormous area in close contact with the capillary blood and is ideally suited for gas exchange.

The gross anatomy of the lower respiratory tract is shown in Fig. 7.

Each lung is covered with a layer of visceral pleura, which is reflected on to the inner surface of the rib cage and diaphragm to form the parietal pleura. Between the visceral and parietal pleura is the pleural space which in normal circumstances contains a little fluid to lubricate the pleura and permit the two layers to move easily over each other. In some diseases the pleural space may contain air, e.g. pneumothorax, or excessive fluid, e.g. pleural effusion.

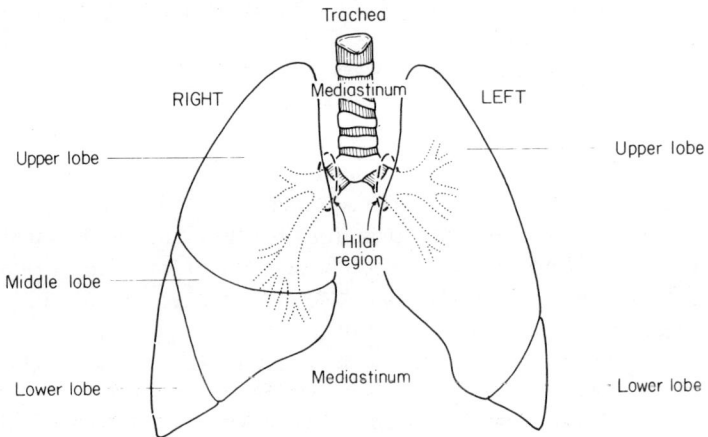

Fig. 7 Gross anatomy of the lower respiratory tract.

The lungs maintain normal and near constant oxygen and carbon dioxide levels in arterial blood. In normal circumstances this is achieved without difficulty because of the efficiency of chest and lung expansion and recoil, the enormity of pulmonary blood flow and the ease of diffusion of gases across the alveolar membranes. Respiration is controlled by chemoreceptors which are present in the brain-stem and peripherally in the carotid and aortic bodies.

Clinical features of respiratory disease

Dyspnoea

Dyspnoea or breathlessness is a subjective awareness of having to increase the rate or effort of respiration. It occurs physiologically during exercise in all people but breathlessness under inappropriate circumstances is a common feature of respiratory disease. It results from either inadequacy of gas transfer at an alveolar level or an increase in the work of respiration, e.g. due to airways obstruction or increased stiffness of the lungs or chest wall.

It is important to remember that dyspnoea can result from non-respiratory disorders such as cardiac failure, anaemia and metabolic acidosis, where the reduction in blood pH is a stimulus to respiration, or in some neuroses (hysterical hyperventilation) where there is no pathological or physiological need to increase respiration.

Cough
This is one of the commonest manifestations of respiratory disease. It results from explosive expiration due to a variety of stimuli, e.g. secretions, irritant dusts, gases, initiating the cough reflex which is an essential means of maintaining airways patency. Cough can be classified as productive or non-productive in terms of sputum.

Sputum
The basis of sputum is mucus which is being produced in excessive quantities by the lining epithelium of the airways. The macroscopic appearance of sputum is variable and can be important clinically.
1. *Mucoid.*   Clear or white appearance indicating excess production of secretions.
2. *Purulent.*   Yellow or greenish colouration due to the presence of micro-organisms, pus and inflammatory products.

Haemoptysis
This is descriptive of blood in the sputum or the production of blood during coughing. It often indicates a sinister lung pathology. The common causes of haemoptysis are:
1. Bronchial carcinoma,
2. Pulmonary thromboembolism,
3. Pulmonary tuberculosis,
4. Lobar pneumonia,
5. Bronchiectasis.

Note. All patients who have haemoptysis require full investigation.

Wheeze
This describes a musical sound most commonly heard in expiration which is indicative of airways narrowing. It is commonly due to asthma or chronic bronchitis but can be localized to a part of one lung where there is partial obstruction of an airway by tumour or following inhalation of a foreign body.

Chest pain
The pain most commonly associated with pulmonary disease is pleuritic chest pain or pleurisy. It occurs when the parietal pleura becomes inflamed and produces a localized, sharp, stabbing pain which is made worse by deep respiration or coughing. If the diaphragmatic pleura is involved it is often referred to the tip of the shoulder. The most likely causes are:
  Pneumonia,
  Pulmonary thromboembolism,
  Bronchial carcinoma,
  Pneumothorax,
  Rib trauma.
Musculoskeletal (chest wall) pain can occur due to rib fracture or intercostal muscle strain as a result of coughing, or trauma. Sharp central chest pain which is aggravated by coughing is often due to tracheitis.

Finger clubbing
This refers to swelling of the terminal phalanges and, less commonly, the toes, due to interstitial oedema and dilation of the small vessels. It occurs in a variety of pulmonary disorders such as:
1. Bronchial carcinoma,
2. Pulmonary or pleural suppuration, e.g. bronchiectasis, lung abscess or empyema,
3. Pulmonary fibrosis, e.g. fibrosing alveolitis, asbestosis.
It can also occur in association with a number of non-pulmonary diseases such as cyanotic congenital heart disease, infective endocarditis, malabsorption syndrome, Crohn's disease, ulcerative colitis and hepatic cirrhosis. In a few cases finger clubbing may be congenital.

Lymph node enlargement
Enlargement of the cervical or axillary lymph nodes may be a feature of some pulmonary disorders such as bronchial carcinoma, pulmonary tuberculosis and sarcoidosis. There are many other non-respiratory causes of lymphadenopathy (p.91 and p.285).

Respiratory tract infections

Upper respiratory tract infections

These are the commonest medical conditions in the UK, accounting for 50% of the total time lost from work. The large majority are viral infections and a wide variety of viruses can produce very similar clinical syndromes. Conversely, a single virus species can produce different clinical syndromes in different individuals.

Common cold syndrome (coryza) is a very well recognized syndrome with increased nasal discharge, sneezing, nasal obstruction and conjunctivitis. There is usually a sore throat, general malaise and chills, but fever is rare. Secondary bacterial infection can occur to produce bronchitis or sinusitis. The syndrome is caused by a number of viruses, including rhinoviruses, parainfluenza viruses, echoviruses, Coxsackie and respiratory synctial virus (RSV).

Pharyngeal syndrome comprises predominantly a sore throat due to inflammation of the pharynx, tonsils and adenoids with cough, hoarseness and cervical lymph node enlargement. General malaise, headache and fever frequently accompany the sore throat. Adenoviruses, influenza viruses, parainfluenza viruses and echoviruses can produce this syndrome but very similar features occur with Group A β-haemolytic streptococcal infection (tonsillitis).

Pharyngoconjunctival syndrome is a variant of the above and is caused by the same virus groups. Conjunctivitis is superimposed on the pharyngitis producing grittiness, photophobia and pain in the eyes.

Influenza syndrome is also well known and although upper respiratory symptoms are usually the presenting features the infection is multi-systemic and systemic upsets are common with fever, chills, generalized aches and pains, loss of appetite, headache and occasionally myocarditis. Symptoms may be mild or very severe and can, in some circumstances, lead to death.

Midwinter epidemics of influenza occur nearly every year, commonly as a result of infection with influenza viruses A or B. *See also* p.201.

Herpangina syndrome is a brief illness due to infection with Coxsackie A virus. It produces vesicles and ulcers in the mouth and gums which can be extremely painful. There may also be associated headache and malaise.

Croup syndrome is a potentially serious condition which predominantly affects young children. It often begins like a common cold but laryngeal obstruction becomes a main feature with inspiratory stridor, breathlessness and, in severe cases, respiratory failure. It is caused by parainfluenza, adenoviruses, influenza and respiratory syncytial viruses and can be associated with *H. influenza* type B infection. In severe cases, tracheostomy may be required to relieve airway obstruction.

Treatment
Most of the above illnesses are self-limiting and in most cases clinical improvement can be expected within a few days. No specific treatments are available although yearly influenza vaccination may be of value in 'at risk' patients with chronic lung disease, etc. Antibiotics are of value if secondary bacterial infection becomes established.

Acute tracheitis and bronchitis
Upper respiratory tract infections can extend into the trachea and bronchi to produce acute tracheitis and bronchitis. This is most likely to occur in influenza, whooping cough or measles infections. Apart from these, the commonest cause is an exacerbation of chronic bronchitis, commonly as a result of *Strep. pneumoniae*, *Strep. pyogenes* or *H. influenzae* infection. Tracheitis produces symptoms of cough, often with little or no sputum, which is often associated with chest pain, but breathlessness is uncommon. Bronchitis is characterized by dyspnoea, wheeze and cough productive of purulent sputum.

Treatment. Cough suppressants may be of value in the treatment of tracheitis but antibiotics are often required in the treatment of bronchitis.

Pneumonias
Pneumonia, or pneumonitis, is an inflammation of the terminal bronchi and alveoli. The pneumonias can be classified on anatomical grounds depending upon whether they are localized in a particular part of the lung (lobar/segmental pneumonia) or whether they are more diffuse (bronchopneumonia). A more useful classification, however, is based on the type of causative agent.

1. Bacterial pneumonias

Pneumococcal pneumonia is caused by *Strep. pneumoniae* and classically presents as a lobar pneumonia with a characteristic clinical picture. There is often an initial upper respiratory tract infection with rapid progression producing general malaise, fever, rigors, dyspnoea and productive cough. The sputum is characteristically 'rusty' in colour. Pleuritic pain is not uncommon and labial herpes simplex is often associated.

Pathologically there is consolidation localized to one lobe resulting in reduced air entry and dullness on percussion of the affected area.

Treatment
Antibiotics: benzyl penicillin is still the treatment of choice
  although resistance to it is increasing,
Oxygen therapy,
Physiotherapy to aid sputum clearance,
Analgesics may be necessary for pleuritic pain.

Staphylococcal pneumonia is less characteristic and more variable in its clinical features, presenting either as a lobar pneumonia, very similar to the above, or as a more diffuse bilateral bronchopneumonia. It tends to affect elderly or debilitated individuals, progressing from an upper respiratory tract infection. Cough, dyspnoea and wheeze are common features and sputum tends to be either yellow or green in colour with occasional flecks of blood. This type of pneumonia may progress to lung abscess formation and pneumothorax may occur.

Treatment. As for pneumococcal pneumonia, although penicillin resistance is more common and flucloxacillin or a cephalosporin might be more appropriate.

Klebsiella pneumonia is frequently found in the bronchopneumonia associated with exacerbation of chronic bronchitis and bronchiectasis. In alcoholics or patients with debilitating disease a severe destructive pneumonia may occur usually affecting the upper lobes. It is difficult to treat as the organism rapidly develops resistance to single antibiotics and combinations containing streptomycin and chloramphenicol may be required.

Haemophilus influenzae pneumonia is a bronchopneumonia which occurs particularly during exacerbations of chronic bronchitis. Most strains are sensitive to ampicillin or cotrimoxazole.

Legionnaire's disease is a pneumonia caused by *Legionella pneumophilia*, a bacterium which has been isolated from water supply tanks and air conditioners of some hotels in recent years. It produces occasional outbreaks of quite severe pneumonia with a significant mortality. It usually responds to erythromycin.

2. *Viral and virus-like pneumonias*

Mild bronchopneumonia frequently occurs with adenovirus, para-influenza virus and rhinovirus infections and more severe pneumonias are well recognized in association with measles, influenza and the respiratory syncytial virus.

Mycoplasma pneumonia, due to the virus-like particle *M. pneumoniae*, can produce quite severe pneumonic symptoms and radiological appearances, often with little to find, other than pyrexia, on examination. It can be treated with antibiotics, e.g. erythromycin or tetracycline.

Psittacosis-ornithosis is a viral-like illness which affects parrots, budgerigars, ducks and pigeons but has also been isolated in a wide variety of domestic, farm and wild animals. It is caused by *Chlamydia psittaci*. Bird fanciers may be affected but more often nowadays there is no clear association with domestic or other birds. The patient infected with the organism may develop either pneumonia, which may be severe with confusion and delirium, or a generalized septicaemic syndrome with pyrexia, malaise, skin rashes and anaemia. The drug of choice is tetracycline.

3. *Pulmonary tuberculosis. See also* p.201.

Tuberculous pneumonia differs from the other pneumonias in a number of important respects. It is characterized by areas of cheese-like necrosis called caseation, parts of which are coughed up leaving holes known as cavities which may cause functional abnormalities even when modern treatment is given. The causal organism, *Mycobacterium tuberculosis*, has a thick protective cell wall which allows the organism to remain dormant for many years either within or without the body until appropriate conditions allow reactivation and growth with the development of a tuberculous lesion. It reproduces itself very slowly which has two consequences:

1. There is a long incubation period of several months allowing travellers returning from endemic areas to enter the country apparently well, only to develop symptoms later.
2. If the organism is not seen on stained smears of sputum or pus, then two or three months may be necessary for it to grow on culture

media followed by a similar time span before its sensitivities to the various anti-tuberculous drugs are known.

If single antibiotics are used in treatment the organism rapidly develops resistance to that medication necessitating initial combination therapy using at least three drugs with modifications once the sensitivities are known.

The tuberculin reaction represents a cell-mediated hypersensitivity reaction to tuberculin protein obtained from the organism when this solution is injected into the superficial layers of the skin. There are three ways of doing the test: Mantoux, Heaf and Tine test, the size of the response giving a useful guide to past or present tuberculous infections. The tests take six to eight weeks to become positive from the time of infection.

Nowadays most infections in Britain are with human organisms which spread by inhalation of infected material from proven cases of pulmonary tuberculosis. Infection has two phases: the primary lesion and post-primary pulmonary tuberculosis.

The primary lesion consists of a small patch of pneumonia with enlargement of the hilar gland draining that area. At this time some organisms may enter the blood and lodge in any other organ leading to disease many years later. The patient may feel slightly unwell for two or three weeks but rarely has any respiratory symptoms. Most primary lesions resolve spontaneously, healing with scarring and calcification which may be seen on chest X-ray many years later.

Post-primary tuberculosis may follow directly from the primary lesion or when an old primary lesion becomes re-activated many years later. The result is a destructive caseating pneumonia usually starting in the upper lobe but spreading to involve both lungs unless treated. The initial stages are insidious, the patient feeling generally unwell with weight loss, lack of energy, night sweats, and a progressively worsening cough with increasing sputum production. Haemoptysis occurs later. At this stage TB organisms may be found in a stained smear of sputum, the tuberculin test is positive and the chest X-ray appearance shows a cavitating pneumonia.

Treatment includes:
1. Isolating the patients while they are infectious,
2. Good anti-tuberculous chemotherapy for sufficient time,
3. Scrupulous contact tracing to identify who is at risk.

Anti-tuberculous chemotherapy. There are several good drugs available for treatment, but in Britain isoniazid and rifampicin form the backbone of most regimes. Both are bactericidal and are usually given in combination for nine months. A third drug, ethambutol or streptomycin, is given for the first three months. Pyrazinamide can be added to the above regime for the first three months when treatment with rifampicin and isoniazid may be reduced to six months. Unless treatment is taken regularly for the appropriate length of time, relapse is likely to occur.

Lung abscess

Lung abscesses are necrotic, suppurative lesions whch develop in the substance of the lung due to infection by pyogenic organisms. They can arise from:
1. Respiratory tract infection,
2. Infection of pulmonary embolism,
3. Inhalation of infected material,
4. Traumatic injury,
5. Extension of infection from below the diaphragm.

Abscess formation is particularly likely to occur if pulmonary infection is inadequately or inappropriately treated, if there is airways constriction, e.g. by bronchial carcinoma or foreign body, or if there has been breakdown of normal defence mechanisms.

When a lung abscess develops there is fever, cough and often a chest ache. After several days patients may cough up a large quantity of foul-smelling sputum. It can be seen as an opacity on chest X-ray which later cavitates, often producing a fluid level.

Treatment. Antibiotics: benzyl penicillin initially followed by oral phenoxymethyl penicillin is effective in most cases although metronidazole may be necessary if anaerobic organisms are present; bronchoscopy and aspiration of secretions; postural drainage; surgery is nowadays rarely necessary.

Bronchiectasis

Pathologically, bronchiectasis is defined as permanent abnormal dilatation of one or more of the larger bronchi resulting from destruction of the elastic supporting tissue within their walls. In the past, whooping cough, measles and tuberculosis were common causes. Mycoplasma and adenoviral infections, cilial dysfunction and immune deficiency states have been implicated. A few cases are congenital.

Sufferers frequently produce varying quantities of mucoid or purulent sputum every day and experience recurrent pneumonic episodes with pleurisy. Haemoptysis is common. Empyema and brain abscesses may occur.

Treatment is of two kinds: medical and surgical.

1. *Medical*
   Regular postural drainage and physiotherapy are essential,
   Treat exacerbations with appropriate antibiotics,
   Long-term prophylactic antibiotics may be given in a few cases.
2. *Surgical*
   If bronchiectasis is localized and symptoms severe, segmental or lobar resection may be curative.

Chronic bronchitis and emphysema
Chronic bronchitis and emphysema are part of a spectrum of clinical conditions which are collectively referred to as *chronic obstructive lung disease*. Most patients suffering from chronic obstructive lung disease have symptoms resulting from a variable mix of the following two categories:

Chronic bronchitis with over-secretion of mucus by glands in the bronchial mucosa presenting as a chronic cough, sputum production particularly in the mornings which may be mucoid or purulent, and increasing dyspnoea eventually leading to respiratory failure.

Emphysema with over-inflation and breakdown of alveoli, resulting in reduction in the overall surface area for gas exchange. Patients often develop dyspnoea with little cough or sputum.

In the initial stages there may be an element of reversible airways obstruction due to mucosal oedema and bronchial muscle spasm although it is usually less marked than that seen in bronchial asthma (less than 10% reversibility). In the later stages the obstruction becomes irreversible resulting from mucous gland hypertrophy, fibrosis and distortions of the bronchi.

Chronic obstructive lung disease is a common cause of death in the UK and there is no doubt that cigarette smoking is the prime causative factor with atmospheric pollution playing a lesser role. There is also some evidence that respiratory infection in infancy may predispose to chronic obstructive lung disease in some individuals. Over the past 15 years the incidence has been gradually falling, probably as a result of the reduction in cigarette consumption and atmospheric pollution.

The frequent symptoms of chronic obstructive lung disease begin insidiously, often with frequent bouts of acute bronchitis. These bouts become more frequent and prolonged until eventually there is no return to normality between attacks. The main symptoms are cough, sputum, wheeze and breathlessness, although only one may predominate. There is usually gradual progression over the years with repeated exacerbations due to acute infection and in some cases respiratory failure develops. In some patients pulmonary arterial hypertension occurs and this can give rise to right heart failure (cor pulmonale, p.40).

Treatment. No treatment is curative but symptomatic improvement can usually be achieved by the following:
1. Stop smoking, reduce atmospheric pollution, avoid dusty atmospheres.
2. Antibiotics: especially useful for the treatment of acute exacerbation and in some patients prophylactic use may be helpful.
3. Bronchodilators, including salbutamol and ipratropium, and occasionally inhaled steroids may be beneficial. Hydrocortisone can be helpful in acute exacerbations but long-term oral corticosteroids should be avoided if possible.
4. Physiotherapy and postural drainage of sputum.
5. Oxygen therapy, particularly during acute exacerbations, although long-term oxygen therapy may be helpful in a few cases if pulmonary hypertension has developed. Controlled levels of oxygen administration are usually necessary (24–35%).
6. Treatment of right heart failure, p.41.

Bronchial asthma
Bronchial asthma is a common condition affecting 5% of the population and characterized by recurrent episodes of generalized airways obstruction which is either partially or completely reversible spontaneously or with the help of drugs. The most prominent features are breathlessness with audible wheeze but in children cough may predominate.

Asthmatic patients appear to have hypersensitive bronchi which can respond to a wide variety of stimuli, some external and some intrinsic, and while one stimulus may predominate in any individual patient, any of the others may cause an attack under appropriate conditions. During attacks there is mucosal swelling with hypersecretion of viscous mucus. There is marked bronchial muscle contraction with muscle hypertrophy developing in longstanding cases. The exact stimulus to an asthmatic attack is often unknown but many of the pathological changes are due to the release of biochemical mediators such as histamine, prostaglandins, bradykinin, leukotrienes, etc.

Causes of asthmatic attacks:
1. Allergy to inhaled material (extrinsic asthma).
   Animal dander,
   Pollens,
   Feathers,
   Mites present in house dust, etc.
2. Upper respiratory tract infections often precipitate attacks, particularly in children.
3. Exercise: 95% of untreated asthmatics wheeze on exercise.
4. Irritants including cigarette smoke, cold damp weather, fumes from paints and petrol, industrial chemicals, e.g. epoxy resins.
5. Aspirin and aspirin-like drugs, i.e. non-steroidal anti-inflammatory drugs.
6. Alcohol, particularly beers and red wine.
7. Stress and emotional trauma (bereavements) may precipitate or aggravate an attack in a patient who already has the disease.
8. No definable cause (intrinsic asthma).

Treatment
For many asthmatics treatment is only necessary during asthmatic attacks, when bronchodilators or systemic steroids are used, but in others prophylactic treatment is required. Several approaches to management are recognized:

Management of precipitating factors. If an allergen can be identified it is obviously helpful if that allergen is avoided. This is often impractical, however, and in many asthmatics the allergens are multiple.

Desensitization is another approach which can be used particularly if a specific, single allergen can be identified. If infection is a known precipitant, a bronchodilator and antibiotic treatment should be given at the onset of symptoms.

Preventative modification of the asthma reaction. Even if it is impossible or impractical to avoid potential causal factors, e.g. allergens, it
is usually possible to prevent or reduce the asthmatic reaction by the
use of preventive medication:
1. *Sodium cromoglycate* is a drug which has been shown to stabilize
   mast cells and prevent release of the biochemical mediators of the
   asthma reaction. The drug, which is only effective if given topically
   by inhalation, has revolutionized the treatment of childhood and
   some allergic asthmas. It has to be taken regularly even when well,
   and may take six to eight weeks to be fully effective. It is of no
   use in an acute attack.
2. *Corticosteroids* act by suppressing the sub-mucosal inflammatory
   response and have a direct smooth muscle relaxant effect. Low dose
   inhaled corticosteroids in the form of beclomethasone (Becotide)
   and betamethasone (Bextasol) taken regularly as a prophylactic
   have revolutionized the treatment of adult intrinsic asthma. Occasionally small daily doses of oral steroids are necessary to effect
   complete control.
   Acute asthma attacks not quickly responding to bronchodilator
   therapy should be treated with corticosteroid; short courses of oral
   steroids, starting with 30–40 mg daily over one to two weeks, may
   be sufficient. In severe attacks requiring hospital admission, initial
   treatment with intravenous hydrocortisone 100–200 mg four to six
   hourly followed by high doses of oral prednisolone reducing over
   one to two weeks may be necessary to control symptoms.

Bronchodilator drugs. Two main types of bronchodilator are used in
clinical practice:
1. β_2-adenoreceptor agonists. These are sympathomimetic drugs
   which act by stimulation of the β_2-adenoreceptors which have
   a selective bronchodilator action. They are preferred to the non-
   selective (β_1 and β_2) agonists because they do not produce
   unwanted cardiac (β_1) stimulation. They are most conveniently given by inhalation, either via a metered dose aerosol or, in
   emergencies, via a nebulizer. The commonly prescribed drugs in
   this group include salbutamol, terbutaline, fenoterol and rimiterol.
   In clinical practice they have several uses:
(a) Taken at the onset of wheezing episodes they often relieve bron-
    chospasm,
(b) Taken before exercise they prevent exercise-induced asthma,
(c) Taken regularly as a mild preventive at the onset of an upper

respiratory tract infection, they may prevent an attack developing,
(d) Taken before preventive medicine (sodium cromoglycate or beclomethasone) they may improve the effects.

Because of their β_1 (cardiac)-adrenoreceptor activity, adrenaline, isoprenaline and orciprenaline are little used nowadays.
2. *Xanthine bronchodilators.* These drugs increase cyclic AMP levels
in bronchial smooth muscle and by this mechanism appear to
reduce bronchospasm. They are available as either oral or parenteral preparations but have a valuable prophylactic role in severe
asthmatics. They are also useful for the prevention of nocturnal
and morning symptoms. The main drugs in this group are theophylline and aminophylline. Side effects are often problematic, e.g.
gastric irritation, palpitations, light-headedness. Because there is
considerable individual variation in the rate of metabolism of xanthine drugs, blood levels are often measured in order to achieve
the optimum dose.

Treatment of severe asthmatic attacks
1. Corticosteroids, given initially as hydrocortisone intravenously
followed by high dose oral prednisolone.
2. Brochodilators: salbutamol, terbutaline, etc., preferably via nebulizer, positive pressure ventilator or intravenous infusion.
3. Oxygen therapy.
4. Intravenous aminophylline if the above measures fail to produce a
rapid improvement. Care must be taken particularly if the patient
has been taking oral xanthine preparations, due to the narrow
therapeutic/toxic serum levels.

Bronchial carcinoma (lung cancer)
The UK has the world's highest incidence and mortality from this
condition. A number of causes are recognized:

Cigarette smoking is the most important factor and it appears that the
lifetime total number of cigarettes smoked correlates best with the
development of lung cancer. Pipe and cigar smoking carry less of a
risk.

Atmospheric pollution is a recognized risk factor and there are distinct
differences in the incidence of the disease between urban and rural
populations.

Industrial factors may be important in some cases, e.g. pitchblende miners (Czechoslovakia), uranium miners (USA), asbestos workers, nickel refiners and haematite workers all have an increased risk of developing lung cancer.

Genetic factors seem to play some part, probably by altering individual susceptibility to carcinogenesis by the other factors. This probably explains why it is that not all heavy smokers, asbestos workers, etc. develop lung cancer.

Pathologically, there are several types of bronchial carcinoma which produce similar clinical features:
1. Squamous cell carcinoma: 45–60%
2. Small cell anaplastic carcinoma (oat cell): 30–40%
3. Adenocarcinoma: 15–20%
4. Large cell anaplastic carcinoma: less than 1%

Features
Many patients are entirely symptom free when the diagnosis is made from a routine chest X-ray. The commonest symptoms are:

Cough. The development of, or worsening of, a dry irritating cough, particularly in a cigarette smoker, should raise the suspicion of bronchial carcinoma. If such a cough persits for more than 3–4 weeks, chest X-ray should be carried out.

Sputum. This may be mucoid or purulent.

Haemoptysis. Variable amounts of blood may be expectorated. This is often the symptom that first brings the patient to the doctor. Any patient who complains of haemoptysis should have a chest X-ray and bronchoscopy if indicated.

Dyspnoea. This tends to be a late symptom and occurs as a result of pulmonary collapse distal to bronchial obstruction. Pleural effusion, diaphragmatic paralysis due to invasion of the phrenic nerves, pneumonia or stiffening of the lungs due to infiltration with tumour may also be responsible in some patients.

Chest pain. Pleuritic chest pain due to spread of tumour to the pleura is the commonest type of pain, but in a few cases a deep central chest ache may be present.

Wheeze or stridor. These are rare symptoms but can occur if there is partial obstruction of the trachea or a major bronchus.

Patients may also complain of general malaise, anorexia and weight loss or have symptoms relating to the presence of metastases in brain, liver, bone, etc. Occasionally bronchial carcinoma produces symptoms that are unrelated to the primary tumour (non-metastatic complications), for example:

Recurrent venous thrombosis,

Hypertrophic pulmonary osteoarthropathy,

Endocrine disorders—Cushing's syndrome, hyperparathyroidism and water intoxication due to hormone production by the tumour cells,

Nephrotic syndrome,

Cerebellar degeneration,

Peripheral neuropathy.

Bronchial carcinoma is diagnosed on the basis of chest X-ray appearances, sputum cytology, bronchoscopic examination and biopsy.

Treatment

Only in the minority of cases (5%), preferably with small peripherally placed tumours and no evidence of secondary spread, can curative surgical treatment be considered. However, even in the most suitable cases the five year post-operative survival is only 20–30%.

Surgery. Resection of part or of a whole lung containing a tumour can be considered if the lesion is localized and the lung function is reasonable.

Radiotherapy. Occasionally a curative course of radiotherapy is given if the tumour is potentially resectable but there is a contra-indication to surgery. More often palliative radiotherapy is used to control troublesome symptoms such as pain, intractable cough, haemoptysis, bronchial obstruction or superior venacaval obstruction.

Chemotherapy. Cytotoxic drugs are the treatment of choice in some cases of small cell anaplastic carcinoma. They are often used in conjunction with radiotherapy to the chest and brain. They are also valuable in the management of malignant pleural effusion.

Symptomatic treatment. Analgesia can be given for pain, antibiotics for infections.

Sarcoidosis

Sarcoidosis is a granulomatous disorder of unknown cause which affects mainly young females. Because of its multisystem involvement it can present in a large number of ways, but the commonest organs affected are the lungs, skin and eyes. Less commonly it involves the gastrointestinal, genitourinary and cardiovascular systems.

In the lung the commonest features are of bilateral lymph node enlargement adjacent to the hila, producing a characteristic X-ray appearance. Occasionally there is a diffuse or patchy involvement of the lung parenchyma producing granulomatous infiltration and fibrosis.

The disease is often associated with pyrexia, general ill health and a reduction in cell-mediated immunity (the finding of a negative skin test to tuberculin is often helpful in making the diagnosis). Occasionally, serum and urinary calcium levels are raised.

The disease may occur acutely and resolve within weeks, and 85–90% of cases settle within 2–3 years. A few cases pursue a relentless course leading to pulmonary fibrosis and respiratory failure.

Treatment. There is no specific treatment but corticosteroids may modify the course of the disease when symptoms are severe.

Occupational lung disease

In some instances the lungs can be damaged as a result of inhalation of dusts, gases or noxious fumes, the exposure occurring during the course of a patient's occupation. A great many varieties of occupational lung disease exist but the commonest in the UK are:
1. Occupational asthma,
2. Coal-workers' pneumoconiosis,
3. Silicosis, e.g. stonemasons, miners, enamellers,
4. Asbestosis, e.g. in builders, dockworkers,
5. Extrinsic allergic alveolitis, e.g. farmers' lung.

A large variety of compounds can be implicated such as iron, barium, tin, mercury, ammonia, sulphur dioxide, oxides of nitrogen, flour (bakers' asthma), mouldy hay (farmers' lung) and sugar cane dust (bagassosis). However, not all personnel exposed to the agent develop lung disease and there are probably a number of contributory factors which determine a patient's susceptibility to the condition.

Occupational asthma or the farmers' lung group of diseases often present with acute symptoms on or within hours of exposure, the patient being better at weekends or when on holiday.

Pneumoconiosis, silicosis and asbestosis have a more insidious onset and X-ray abnormalities may precede the appearance of symptoms. Thereafter, there is a progressive fibrosis of the lungs over a variable period, producing breathlessness as a result of reduced lung elasticity, thickening of alveolar septa and obstruction of airways. These patients suffer recurrent bouts of superimposed infection and eventually respiratory failure may develop. In asbestosis the risk of developing bronchial carcinoma or a malignant pleural tumour (mesothelioma) is greatly increased.

Treatment
1. Removal from exposure to the causal agent is essential in occupational asthma and extrinsic allergic alveolitis.
2. Prevention of pneumoconiosis, e.g. silicosis and asbestosis, by the use of face-masks, respirators, extraction of dusts, etc. is the only effective approach.

Pulmonary thromboembolic disease
Pulmonary thromboembolic disease refers to a combination of:
1. Thrombosis, often within the peripheral veins of the lower limbs or the large veins of the pelvis.
2. Embolization of the clot from the site of formation to the lung via the vena cava, right heart and pulmonary arteries.
Pulmonary thromboembolism is a common cause of death especially after major surgery or post-natally. It can also occur in association with the use of the contraceptive pill and in a variety of malignant diseases.

Deep venous thrombosis
This is probably quite a common condition and passes unnoticed in a large number of instances. The stimulus to intravascular thrombosis (which occurs most commonly in the deep veins of the lower limbs) is probably a combination of factors including:
Relative stasis of venous blood,
Increased coagulability of blood, e.g. during stress, contraceptive pill,
Minor damage to the walls of the veins.
Classically the development of deep venous thrombosis produces pain, swelling and tenderness in the calf with extension up to the groin in a

few cases. In an unknown percentage of cases part of the blood clot passes to the lungs producing pulmonary embolization.

Pulmonary embolization

A single small pulmonary embolus is functionally relatively unimportant, producing transient mild dyspnoea, pleuritic chest pain and occasional haemoptysis. A single large embolus or recurrent small emboli can lead to significant functional impairment by causing imbalance of pulmonary ventilation and perfusion, producing marked dyspnoea. Recurrent small emboli over several months or years can present as exercise-induced dyspnoea and fatigue due to hypoxia and may eventually lead to pulmonary arterial hypertension.

When massive pulmonary embolism occurs, the right and left pulmonary arteries may become obstructed by a 'saddle' embolus with marked reduction in cardiac output. If the pulmonary artery occlusion is complete, death rapidly ensues, but if the occlusion is incomplete the clot may either break up with the fragments passing distally into the branches of the pulmonary artery or require urgent medical removal or dissolution with intravenous streptokinase.

Diseases of the pleura

Pneumothorax

Pneumothorax is the presence of air in the pleural cavity and results from the presence of a hole in the parietal or visceral pleura. When this occurs the lung on the affected side collapses away from the chest wall and does not expand on inspiration. The causes are:
1. *Spontaneous.* This is the commonest type, usually occurring in fit young males with no history of pulmonary disease. It is thought to be due to the bursting of small apical subpleural congenital cysts.
2. *Trauma.* Penetrating chest injuries or rib fractures can, by tearing the parietal and/or the visceral pleura, produce pneumothorax.
3. *Obstructive lung disease.* Chronic bronchitis and emphysema are frequently associated with the development of lung cysts or bullae which can rupture into the pleural space.
4. *Bronchial carcinoma.* When a pneumothorax develops there is usually pleuritic pain on the affected side and dyspnoea which may be out of proportion to the degree of lung collapse. In some cases the patient becomes agitated, hypotensive, shocked and eventually loses consciousness. When this occurs it suggests increasing pres-

sure within the pneumothorax (tension pneumothorax) due to a ball-valve effect leading to shift of the mediastinum and compression of the large veins of the chest, causing occlusion of the venous return to the heart (p.8).

Treatment. No treatment is required for a small pneumothorax (less than 20% lung collapse) when complete resolution usually occurs within four weeks.

With a large pneumothorax, bilateral pneumothorax or tension pneumothorax, an intercostal chest drain has to be inserted and may be life-saving. This is passed through the chest wall into the pleural space, the other end being attached to a valve mechanism, e.g. under water, allowing the lung to re-expand.

In a few cases pneumothorax is a recurrent problem, when an irritant material may be put into the pleural space to promote fusion of the parietal and visceral pleura. If this is unsuccessful an operation may be necessary to remove the pleura and allow the lung to stick to the chest wall.

Pleural effusion

Pleural effusion is an accumulation of fluid in the pleural space and results from either transudation or exudation from the pleural surfaces. It is not a disease in its own right but a feature of some underlying disease. If the accumulation of fluid produces significant compression of the lung then the patient complains of breathlessness. Pleuritic pain or ache over the affected area frequently occurs.

A large number of causes are recognized:
1. Congestive cardiac failure,
2. Bronchial carcinoma or secondary lung tumours,
3. Infections, e.g. pneumonia or pulmonary TB,
4. Pulmonary infarction,
5. Primary pleural tumours, e.g. mesothelioma,
6. Connective tissue disorders,
7. General hypoproteinaemic states,
8. Myxoedema,
9. Pancreatitis.

Treatment. Treatment of the underlying disease often leads to disappearance of the effusion. If the effusion is large and breathlessness is a problem, the fluid can be removed by the insertion of an intercostal needle or drain, taking care not to allow air to enter the pleural space.

Empyema
Empyema is a purulent pleural effusion. It was a relatively common
condition in the pre-antibiotic era but is now relatively rare. It can
result from extension of an infective pulmonary lesion, e.g. pneumonia, lung abscess, bronchiectasis or pulmonary TB, to the pleural
space, or occur as part of a generalized septicaemia. Nowadays it is
most commonly associated with penetrating chest injuries or thoracic
surgery.
An acute empyema presents with features of a pleural effusion and
associated pyrexia and leucocytosis. In chronic empyema the features
may be less obvious with general ill health, finger clubbing and the
occasional development of a sinus through the chest wall.

Treatment. If the pus is thin it can be drained through a large bore
intercostal chest drain but if thick, surgical intervention is usually
required.
Antibiotics often have to be given over prolonged periods (6–8
weeks for pyogenic infections, 9–18 months for tuberculosis).

Respiratory failure
If the lungs are unable to maintain adequate gas exchange, and hypoxia with an arterial oxygen tension (Pa_{O_2}) of less than 60 mmHg
results, then respiratory failure is said to have occurred. Two types
of respiratory failure are recognized:
Type 1. If the arterial carbon dioxide tension (Pa_{CO_2}) is normal or
        low,
Type 2. If the arterial carbon dioxide tension is above 50 mmHg.

Note. Occasionally there is a reduction in arterial oxygen concentrations without any significant respiratory failure. This occurs in patients
with right to left intracardiac shunts due to longstanding atrial or
ventricular septal defects.

Acute type 1 respiratory failure
In this type the hypoxia usually triggers reflex hyperventilation and
carbon dioxide is blown off, so reducing the arterial carbon dioxide
tension. Three pathophysiological mechanisms may produce the hypoxia:
1. An increase in the physiological shunt of desaturated blood from
   the right to the left side of the heart, i.e. in a pneumonia blood

flows through alveoli filled with pus and no gas exchange takes place.
2. Increased alveolar-capillary block, i.e. an increase in the thickness of the alveolar wall impairing gas exchange, e.g. pulmonary oedema from left ventricular failure.
3. Ventilation perfusion imbalance—when well-ventilated areas are poorly perfused and vice versa, e.g. an acute asthma attack.
This type of respiratory failure is found in:
Pulmonary infection,
Acute asthmatic attacks,
Acute left vetricular failure,
Pulmonary thromboembolism,
Adult respiratory distress syndrome (p.9).

Treatment is directed towards relieving the underlying cause. As the carbon dioxide tension is normal or low, it is quite safe to use high concentrations of inspired oxygen (60%) to relieve the hypoxia.

Acute type 2 respiratory failure
This type occurs whenever alveolar ventilation is inadequate to blow off carbon dioxide which accumulates in the blood. There are two primary causes:
1. Abnormalities of the respiratory centre and the neuromuscular and skeletal afferent pathways of respiration.
2. Deficiencies in the chemo-regulatory centres of the brain-stem and carotid bodies.
The respiratory centre may be depressed following head injury and during anaesthesia, drug overdose and alcohol intoxication. The afferent nerves may be affected by infections such as poliomyelitis and diphtheria and the Guillain–Barré syndrome while myasthenia gravis affects the nerve/muscle endplate. In severe chest injuries a flail segment of chest wall impairs ventilation. Management of these cases involves intermittent positive pressure ventilation until the underlying condition resolves spontaneously or with treatment.

While in normal subjects the sensitive chemoreceptors of the brain-stem and carotid bodies respond quickly to changes in arterial carbon dioxide tension so maintaining the blood gases within normal limits, in a chronic bronchitic response to carbon dioxide may be impaired and the respiratory drive becomes dependent on the degree of hypoxia, a less sensitive mechanism which allows the build-up of carbon dioxide within the body. This situation becomes more marked in acute exacerbations of chronic bronchitis. Under these circumstances it is dangerous to give high concentrations of inspired oxygen as this interferes with the hypoxic respiratory drive allowing the carbon dioxide to rise to dangerous levels. Supplementary oxygen should be given in a controlled way using masks, giving 24, 28 or 35%, the exact level depending on repeated blood gas estimations. It may be necessary to give a respiratory stimulant, e.g. nikethamide or doxapram, along with controlled oxygen during the early stages of treatment of an acute exacerbation. Physiotherapy and antibiotics are necessary to treat any infection while nebulized bronchodilators, usually salbutamol or terbutaline and ipratropium bromide, help to relieve bronchospasm. Sedation should be avoided as it further depresses the respiratory centre.

Chronic respiratory failure
Chronic type 1 respiratory failure may occur in fibrotic lung disease, e.g. asbestosis, while some patients with chronic bronchitis may have both hypoxia and raised carbon dioxide levels, type 2 failure, even when at their best.

Treatment is directed towards controlling the underlying disease with appropriate oxygen supplementation.

Inhalation of foreign bodies
The inhalation of foreign matter into the trachea and bronchial system is always a serious and potentially fatal situation. In normal individuals it usually occurs accidentally but certain medical conditions may predispose to its occurrence:
1. Depressed 'gag' reflex, e.g. local anaesthetics,
2. Depressed pharyngeal and laryngeal reflexes, e.g. CNS disorders affecting the brain-stem, such as polio, multiple sclerosis or motor neurone disease (bulbar palsy), or cerebrovascular disease (pseudo-bulbar palsy),
3. Drug-induced CNS depression, e.g. anaesthetic agents, analgesic, opiate, benzodiazepine, antidepressant or alcohol overdosage,
4. Coma.
The inhaled material may be solid (food, peanuts, teeth , bone, dental materials) or liquid (vomit, blood, water).
   Solid material usually produces airways obstruction, sometimes leading to significant lung collapse and infection. Vegetable material

is highly irritant, producing intense local reaction with a progressive distal pneumonia. The apical segment of the right lower lower lobe is most commonly affected.

Inhaled liquid material tends to produce a more generalized bronchopneumonia.

Inhalation of foreign matter should be suspected in any individual who chokes and then develops an unexplained cough, wheeze, breathlessness and occasionally haemoptysis. The condition is particularly serious in young children because the airways are much smaller in diameter.

Prevention
1. In general, it is very important to prevent inhalation of foreign material from the mouth.
2. General anaesthesia (GA) should not be administered within 4 hours of eating and drinking.

If the patient is known to have depressed 'gag' or cough reflexes, he should:
(a) Not be given GA within 12 hours of eating and drinking,
(b) Be given a GA only if an endotracheal tube has been passed and the cuff inflated,
(c) Be nursed in the prone position with regular aspiration of secretions.

Note. If there is any doubt as to whether or not inhalation has occurred, a chest X-ray is mandatory.

Treatment. In acute choking episodes good results can be achieved by applying the Heimlich manoeuvre. This is performed by approaching the patient from behind, passing the arms around his waist and rapidly compressing his epigastrium. This often produces a bout of coughing with expulsion of the foreign matter (p. 7).

If the foreign material becomes lodged in the bronchial tree, a rigid bronchoscope should be passed under general anaesthesia. Any liquid should be aspirated while solid material may be removed using special forceps. If vegetable material has produced a significant local reaction, antibiotics and corticosteroids may be given and the bronchoscopy repeated within a few days. Thoracotomy may be required if bronchoscopic removal is unsuccessful.

6 Anaemia, polycythaemia, haemorrhagic disorders and anticoagulants

Anaemia

Anaemia signifies a reduction in the concentration of haemoglobin in the peripheral blood, below the normal for the age and sex of the patient. In adults, it is present when the haemoglobin concentration is less than 13.0 g/dl in men, or 11.5 g/dl in women. In childhood, the haemoglobin concentration is high at birth and then falls to a level below the normal adult value during childhood, increasing to the adult range at puberty.

In anaemia, because of the reduced amount of haemoglobin, the oxygen-carrying power of the blood is reduced. This hypoxaemia accounts for the symptoms and signs. The severity of the symptoms depends partly on the level of haemoglobin and partly on the rate of development of the anaemia. These symptoms include fatigue, muscular weakness, breathlessness on exertion and palpitations. Pallor of the skin may be apparent but this is a most unreliable sign. Moderate anaemia may be present without obvious skin pallor and not all subjects who look pale are anaemic. Pallor of the mucous membranes of the mouth and of the conjunctivae is a more reliable sign of anaemia, but this also must be interpreted with caution. The only certain proof of anacmia is estimation of the haemoglobin concentration in the blood.

Angina may occur with the onset of anaemia in patients with pre-existing mild coronary artery disease. Congestive cardiac failure may occur in association with severe anaemia, especially in older patients and in those who already have cardiac disease. These clinical features are similar in any type of anaemia. It is important to distinguish symptoms and signs due to the anaemia from those of the disease causing it, e.g. the symptoms of carcinoma of the stomach which caused a blood-loss anaemia.

In all cases, anaemia is due to one of three general causes—loss of red cells from the body, i.e. haemorrhage, destruction of red cells within the body, i.e. haemolysis, or failure to make normal red cells in adequate number, i.e. impairment of erythropoiesis in the bone marrow.

Important types of anaemia
1. Iron deficiency,
2. Megaloblastic,
3. Haemolytic,
4. Aplastic or hypoplastic,
5. Anaemia of chronic disorder.

Iron deficiency anaemia
When there is an inadequate amount of iron available for haemoglobin synthesis, erythrocytes are produced which are deficient in haemo-globin (hypochromic) and smaller than normal (microcytic). The typical anaemia of chronic iron deficiency is therefore described as *hypochromic microcytic anaemia*.

The average loss of iron from the body, following the desquamation of epithelium from the skin and renal and alimentary tracts, is only about 1 mg daily. The only other way in which iron is lost from the body is by loss of blood. It follows that the daily iron requirement of healthy male adults is about 1 mg. During the years that menstruation is occurring, the normal female is obviously losing iron periodically and expressed as an average replacement requirement this amounts to about 2 mg daily. Pregnancy increases further the iron requirement. As the average diet in Britain contains about 15 mg iron and as only about 10% of ingested iron is absorbed, it is not surprising that iron deficiency is common in women, especially during pregnancy and in those with heavy menstrual loss. In men, iron deficiency is uncommon unless there is bleeding.

It is always necessary to find the cause of iron deficiency, as it may be a condition requiring urgent treatment, e.g. carcinoma of the bowel. The most important cause of iron deficiency anaemia is loss of blood, as in menorrhagia (heavy menstrual loss) or gastrointestinal bleeding from peptic ulcer or carcinoma. Iron deficiency may result from nutritional inadequacy, especially in the elderly. The main sources of iron in the diet are meat and green vegetables. The third possible cause of iron deficiency is malabsorption, as in coeliac disease or following gastrectomy.

The symptoms and signs of iron deficiency anaemia are the general clinical features of anaemia, but associated in some cases with signs of the underlying disease that has caused it. In addition, in some patients with longstanding severe iron deficiency, changes occur in epithelial tissues. The nails may become flattened, or in severe cases, concave and spoon-shaped—koilonychia. Atrophic glossitis causes a pale, smooth tongue, sometimes associated with attacks of painful burning sensation when the tongue may show red areas of inflammation. Angular stomatitis may develop with painful red cracks at the angles of the mouth. In a few patients with longstanding iron deficiency, dysphagia develops due to a band of epithelial tissue obstructing the oesophagus (post-cricoid web). This condition, known as the Plummer–Vinson or Patterson–Kelly syndrome, is associated with an increased incidence of post-cricoid carcinoma.

In the treatment of iron deficiency anaemia, iron is given in the form of tablets of ferrous sulphate. Ferrous salts are unstable in solution and liquid preparations are rarely used except in the treatment of young children; solutions of iron salts tend to stain the teeth. In a few patients who cannot take oral iron preparations, who have severe malabsorption or who have continuing blood loss, iron may have to be given by injection. The patient with severe anaemia resulting from blood loss may require blood transfusion (p.24)

Megaloblastic anaemia
This type of anaemia is characterized by the presence in the bone marrow of abnormal nucleated red cell precursors, called megaloblasts. These cells differ from the normal nucleated red cell precursors (normoblasts) in being larger and having an abnormal appearance of the chromatin network of the nucleus. In the peripheral blood, the red cells are larger than normal (macrocytosis) and usually the numbers of leucocytes and platelets are moderately reduced. Megaloblastic anaemia results from impairment of DNA synthesis caused by deficiency of either vitamin B_{12} or folic acid. In patients with vitamin B_{12} deficiency, in addition to the haematological changes there may be neurological manifestations due to damage to the peripheral nerves and to the posterior and lateral columns of the spinal cord (subacute combined degeneration of the cord). The usual symptoms are paraesthesiae in the hands and feet and weakness of the legs with unsteadiness in walking. Glossitis is common with episodes of a painful red tongue followed by atrophy of the papillae and a pale shiny, smooth tongue.

The principal causes of vitamin B_{12} deficiency are:
1. *Pernicious anaemia.* An autoimmune disorder, in which there is atrophy of gastric mucosal cells. This leads to achlorhydria and

also lack of intrinsic factor with consequent failure of absorption of vitamin B_{12}.

2. *Gastrectomy*. Partial or total, with resulting inadequate production of intrinsic factor.

3. *Disease of terminal ileum,* e.g. Crohn's (inflammatory) disease. Vitamin B_{12} is absorbed at that site; disease of this area may thereby cause malabsorption of the vitamin (p.119).

4. *'Blind-loop' syndrome*. Where there are by-passed loops of small intestine, as a result of disease or previous surgery, in which abnormal proliferation of bacteria occurs, which compete with the host for vitamin B_{12}.

5. *Nutritional*. Uncommon in western Europe. Vitamin B_{12} is present mainly in food of animal origin.

The treatment of megaloblastic anaemia due to vitamin B_{12} deficiency is by regular intramuscular injections of hydroxycobalamin, usually for the rest of the patient's life.

The principal causes of *folic acid deficiency* are:

(a) *Nutritional*. Folic acid is present in many foods of vegetable and animal origin, e.g. green vegetables, liver. Deficiency is relatively common, especially in elderly people taking a poor diet.

(b) *Malabsorption*. Coeliac disease.

(c) *Increased requirement*. Pregnancy, malignant disease.

(d) *Drugs*, e.g. the anticonvulsant phenytoin.

The treatment of megaloblastic anaemia due to folic acid deficiency is with tablets of folic acid.

Haemolytic anaemia

This type of anaemia is caused by abnormal destruction of red cells within the body and consequent reduction in the average red cell lifespan. The clinical features of haemolytic anaemia are those of anaemia and, usually, jaundice due to the increased rate of haemoglobin breakdown. The spleen frequently becomes enlarged in patients with haemolytic anaemia. Haemolytic anaemia is due to either (1) a defect in the red cell or (2) to the development of an abnormal haemolytic mechanism.

Red cell defect. One example is *congenital spherocytosis*, a familial condition in which the red cells are abnormally spherical and are prematurely destroyed in the spleen. Splenectomy completely stops the abnormal haemolytic process although the red cells retain their spherical shape. *Congenital deficiency of the red cell enzyme glucose-6-phosphate dehydrogenase (G-6-P-D)* results in impaired defence of the red cell against oxidative destruction. As a result a large number of chemical substances, including many drugs, provoke a haemolytic episode in such subjects. This enzyme deficiency occurs most commonly in people of Mediterranean or African origin. Sickle cell disease is another example.

Abnormal haemolytic mechanism. In autoimmune haemolytic anaemia, antibodies are present in the serum or on the surface of the red cells. In most such cases remissions can be obtained by prednisolone therapy. Sometimes prolonged steroid therapy is necessary to maintain remission, and splenectomy is of value in some of these cases. A similar type of autoimmune haemolytic anaemia may occur as a secondary feature in patients with lymphoma and chronic lymphatic leukaemia.

A number of drugs may cause haemolytic anaemia. Apart from G-6-P-D deficiency already referred to, drugs may cause haemolysis by a direct toxic action on normal red cells or as a result of the development of an abnormal immunological mechanism, e.g. methyldopa, one of the older anti-hypertensive drugs (p.47).

Aplastic or hypoplastic anaemia
This results from a reduction in the amount of functionally effective haemopoietic tissue in the marrow. Usually the precursor cells of the granulocytes and platelets are affected as well as those of the red cells so that the peripheral blood shows a reduction in the red cells, leucocytes and platelets, i.e. *pancytopenia. Leucopenia,* when severe, greatly increases the susceptibility to severe infections and thrombocytopenia causes an abnormal bleeding tendency.

Aplastic anaemia results from toxic damage to the bone marrow from chemical agents, including drugs and physical agents such as ionizing radiation. Certain drugs, e.g. cytotoxic agents, regularly produce marrow depression in all subjects. Other drugs cause marrow damage only very occasionally, apparently as a result of idiosyncrasy or hypersensitivity of the patient. Drugs in therapeutic use which occasionally cause aplastic anaemia include sulphonamides, chloramphenicol, phenylbutazone and indomethacin.

In some cases, drug toxicity affects only leucocyte production— *agranulocytosis*—and in others, only the platelets may be involved —*thrombocytopenia.*

The patient with severe aplastic anaemia may require repeated blood transfusions to maintain an acceptable haemoglobin level and if serious bleeding is occurring due to thrombocytopenia, platelet transfusions are also required. The reduced resistance to infections associated with severe leucopenia requires energetic antibiotic treatment of any suspected infection.

Anaemia resulting from impaired production of red cells in the bone marrow also occurs in primary marrow disease, e.g. the myeloid leukaemias, myelofibrosis and myeloma.

Anaemia of chronic disorder

Anaemia occurs in association with a variety of chronic disease processes, in particular, chronic infections, malignancy and the collagen disorders, e.g. rheumatoid arthritis. The red cells are usually normocytic and normochromic or sometimes slightly hypochromic. The anaemia responds only to the succesful treatment of the underlying disorder.

In chronic renal failure a normochromic, normocytic anaemia is almost invariable; it responds only if the renal failure can be relieved.

Polycythaemia

Polycythaemia means an abnormally large number of red cells in the circulating blood. This causes a high red cell count, high haematocrit and usually also high haemoglobin concentration. In *true, or absolute polycythaemia* these increased values result from an increase above normal in the total mass of circulating red cells. A high red cell count, haematocrit or haemoglobin may also occur due to haemoconcentration, when there is a reduction in the plasma volume. This is referred to as *relative or spurious polycythaemia* and may occur acutely in dehydration or more chronically without obvious explanation. The only way to distinguish true from relative polycythaemia is by measurement of the total circulating red cell volume, using radiochromium as a red cell label in an isotope tracer dilution technique.

True polycythaemia may be primary, due to a proliferative disorder in the bone marrow, or secondary, due to disease elsewhere.

In *primary polycythaemia* all the cells of the marrow are usually involved so that the leucocyte count and platelet count are increased as well as the red cell count. Splenomegaly is present in over 50% of cases. The typical patient with severe polycythaemia has a florid, high coloured face and congestion of the vessels of the mucous membranes of the mouth and the conjunctiva. Because of the increased number of cells, the viscosity of the blood is increased which contributes to the high risk of thrombotic complications: venous thrombosis, cerebral infarction, myocardial infarction. Paradoxically there is also, frequently, an increased bleeding tendency. One reason for this is that the platelets, although increased in numbers, may be functionally incompetent. Treatment of primary polycythaemia is by venesection with removal of blood and, in severe cases, radioactive phosphorus which depresses marrow activity by irradiation.

Secondary polycythaemia is usually due to a compensatory increase in erythropoiesis as a result of tissue hypoxia. Thus, the most common causes are chronic pulmonary disease and cyanotic congenital heart disease. Secondary polycythaemia also may result from excess erythropoietin, inappropriately produced by a tumour, e.g. hypernephroma or hepatoma. The treatment of secondary polycythaemia is that of the underlying disorder. When the polycythaemia is very severe, and the blood viscosity high, venesections may be required to reduce the risk of thrombosis.

Haemorrhagic disorders
Normally a balance is achieved between the physiological processes which maintain the circulating blood in a fluid condition, without thrombosis occurring, and those processes which allow prompt cessation of haemorrhage when blood escapes from the vascular system. The coagulation process, leading to fibrin production, is balanced by the fibrinolytic process by which fibrin is broken down. When the vascular endothelium is damaged, platelets adhere and release adenine nucleotides and serotonin, which set off the process leading to coagulation and haemostasis. Platelet aggregation occurs and fibrin formation results from the series of reactions of the coagulation Factors I–XII. Inadequate activity of one or more of these factors, a deficiency of platelets, or an abnormality of the blood vessels may result in impairment of the haemostatic mechanism and consequently an increased tendency to bleed.

Coagulation factor defects
1. *Hereditary disorders* include *haemophilia A* (Factor VIII deficiency), *Christmas disease* (haemophilia B, Factor IX deficiency) and *von Willebrand's disease.*
2. *Acquired coagulation disorders.* The most common causes are liver disease and the effect of anticoagulant drugs.

Haemophilia and Christmas disease. Although these are different hereditary disorders due to deficiency of different coagulation factors, the mode of inheritance and the clinical features of the two disorders are the same.

Both are conditions inherited as sex-linked recessive characters, the genes for the abnormalities being carried on the X-chromosome. All the daughters of an affected male are carriers but his sons are normal. The children of a carrier female have an equal chance of being normal or affected (if male), or normal or carrier (if female). Female carriers usually have no bleeding tendency.

The clinical features include:
1. Excessive bleeding after trauma, including surgery. Haemorrhage after dental extraction is almost invariable and may be severe and prolonged.
2. Deep muscle haematomata occurring either spontaneously or after trivial trauma.
3. Haemarthroses. Painful haemorrhage into joints. If repeated many times, ultimately lead to severe joint damage and crippling.
4. Haematuria.
5. Bleeding into and from the intra-oral soft tissues after trivial trauma.

Note. Haematomata of the tongue or floor of the mouth are potentially dangerous and they may extend rapidly.

The treatment of a haemorrhagic episode is to raise the plasma level of Factor VIII or IX by intravenous injections of concentrate of the appropriate Factor—VIII in haemophilia A, IX in Christmas disease. A severe haemophiliac may have a Factor VIII level of less than 1% normal. In treatment of a haemarthrosis, sufficient Factor VIII is injected to maintain the patient's plasma level to at least 30% for several days. In a more severe haemorrhage or to cover bleeding from surgery, the plasma level would be raised to 50–100%. Concentrates of Factors VIII and IX are prepared from human plasma at the plasma fractionation centres for use within the National Health Service; they are also available commercially. Cryoprecipitate is a relatively crude extract containing Factor VIII, but not Factor IX, and prepared locally in blood transfusion departments.

The use of human blood products carries a slight risk of transmission of viral hepatitis and recently there has also been concern about the possible transmission of the acquired immune deficiency syndrome (AIDS). Methods of preparation of plasma concentrates, e.g. heat treatment, are being developed with the aim of minimizing or eliminating this danger.

Because of the danger of haemorrhage following dental extraction, all persons suffering from an increased bleeding tendency should be strongly advised to have adequate and regular dental examination and conservation. When dental extraction is required, this should be arranged in collaboration with a physician experienced in the management of haemophilia and bleeding disorders. Usually this will be a physician on the staff of the nearest haemophilia centre. All persons suffering from an hereditary bleeding disorder should be registered at the haemophilia centre nearest their home, where details of their haematological condition should be available.

When dental extraction is to be carried out, it is usual to minimize the requirement for factor replacement by giving an antifibrinolytic agent—aminocaproic acid (EACA, Epsikapron) or tranexamic acid (Cyklokapron). Using tranexamic acid, 1 g is given by slow intravenous injection prior to surgery and thereafter 1 g orally four times daily for 5 days. If haematuria is present this procedure should be cancelled to avoid the danger of ureteric blockage by clots. Patients with severe haemophilia A or Christmas disease should have their levels of Factor VIII or IX raised to about 50% by injections of the appropriate factor. Twice daily injections may be required for 3–4 days. In patients with mild haemophilia, an alternative therapy, to avoid giving blood products, is the use of desmopressin (DDAVP). This has the effect of boosting Factor VIII concentrations. DDAVP is of no value in severe haemophilia. Infection delays wound healing and predisposes to prolonged bleeding. Patients should be given penicillin V 500 mg orally four times daily for 7 days as prophylaxis. Erythromycin is used if the patient is allergic to pencillin.

Intramuscular injections should never be given to those with coagulation factor deficiencies because of the danger of haematoma formation. Aspirin and probably all non-steroidal anti-inflammatory drugs should be avoided because of the possibility of gastric bleeding. Paracetamol, dihydrocodeine or pentazocine are satisfactory analgesics.

Von Willebrand's disease. This disorder is inherited as an autosomal dominant character and affects both sexes. The bleeding tendency is usually mild and consists of easy bruising, epistaxes and excessive bleeding after minor injuries or surgery, including dental extractions. There is reduction in the plasma Factor VIII activity and also a functional defect of platelets. In treatment of a bleeding episode, desmopressin (DDAVP) may be used, or in more severe bleeding, cryoprecipitate injected as a source of Factor VIII.

Thrombocytopenia

The lower border of the normal range of platelet counts is usually taken as $150 \times 10^9/l$. A platelet count less than this indicates thrombocytopenia. Spontaneous bleeding usually does not occur unless the platelet count is less than $40 \times 10^9/l$. The clinical features of the bleeding tendency due to thrombocytopenia include easy bruising, spontaneous haemorrhages in the skin and mucous membranes, epistaxis, bleeding gums and excessive haemorrhage from trauma or surgery. The skin haemorrhages include both multiple tiny dot haemorrhages (petechiae) and larger haemorrhagic areas (ecchymoses).

Thrombocytopenia may be *primary, idiopathic thrombocytopenic purpura*, due to the development of auto-antibodies to platelets. Treatment is by prednisolone and, in some cases, splenectomy. Occasionally, if there is severe bleeding, a platelet transfusion is given and blood transfusion may be required if there is considerable loss of blood.

Secondary thrombocytopenia occurs due to drug toxicity, hypersplenism with destruction of platelets in a greatly enlarged spleen, or disease of the bone marrow, e.g. leukaemia, myeloma or aplastic anaemia. Treatment in secondary thrombocytopenia consists or removing the cause or relieving the underlying disorder, if possible.

Vascular haemorrhagic disorders

The haemorrhagic tendency due to vascular disorders is usually relatively mild and consists of purpura, or bleeding into the skin—petechiae and ecchymoses. The commonest associations of this type of purpura are old age, severe infections, drug toxicity, Cushing's disease, adrenocortical steroid therapy and scurvy (vitamin C deficiency). *Henoch–Schonlein or anaphylactoid purpura* is a hypersensitivity reaction usually to bacteria but sometimes to a drug or food. In addition to the skin haemorrhages, particularly over the buttocks, joint pains and vomiting, diarrhoea and abdominal colic are common.

Hereditary haemorrhagic telangiectasia (Osler–Rendu–Weber disease) affects both sexes and is transmitted as a simple dominant characteristic. The telangiectases consist of small masses of dilated capillaries and arterioles, most frequently in the skin and the mucous membranes of the nose and mouth but sometimes in the gastrointestinal tract or other organs. The lesions increase in number and size as the subject gets older. The commonest bleeding manifestation is epistaxis, which may be frequent and persistent and lead to chronic iron deficiency anaemia.

Anticoagulant drugs

These drugs are used to prevent thrombus formation or to limit the extension of an existing thrombus. There are two types of anticoagulant drugs: (a) direct acting, which must be given by injection, e.g. heparin; (b) indirect acting, given orally, e.g. warfarin.

Heparin is a mucopolysaccharide which has an immediate inhibitory effect on several stages of the clotting process and so prevents coagulation. It is active *in vitro* as well as *in vivo*. Heparin must be given by injection, usually intravenous, for therapeutic effect but subcutaneous heparin is also now being used in an attempt to provide prophylaxis against thrombosis. Intravenous heparin therapy is given preferably by continous infusion, but can also be given by intermittent injections at intervals of not more than 6 hours. When continuous heparin therapy is being given, the correctness of the dose can be checked by the whole blood clotting time or the activated partial thromboplastin time.

The main adverse effect of heparin is haemorrhage. If minor in degree, it is only neccessary to stop heparin administration as the duration of action is only 4–6 hours. If major haemorrhage occurs the anticoagulant effect of heparin can be neutralized immediately by an intravenous injection of protamine sulphate. Allergic reactions and thrombocytopenia occasionally occur as a result of heparin injections.

Warfarin is the oral anticoagulant most commonly used in the UK. It is one of the coumarin group of drugs of which several have been used as anticoagulants. Warfarin interferes with the formation of clotting Factors II, VII, IX and X from vitamin K in the liver. As it has no immediate effect on the clotting factors already circulating in the plasma, there is a delay of 48–72 hours before a full anticoagulant effect is produced. Thereafter the daily dosage is determined depending on the result of the prothrombin time or thrombotest. Prolongation of the prothrombin time to between two and three times the normal value or a thrombotest result of 5–15% activity is regarded as satisfactory anticoagulant effect. Prothrombin times less than twice the normal value or a thrombotest result of more than 15% activity indicate inadequate anticoagulation, whereas prothrombin times more than three times normal or a thrombotest result of less than 5% activity indicate excessive anticoagulation. All patients on anticoagulants should have a card giving details of the reason for this therapy, the name of the drug and its dosage, as well as the most recent and other previous coagulation test results. As there is considerable individual variation in dose required it is essential that one of these tests is carried out regularly and frequently, as excessive dosage produces a serious risk of haemorrhage. Bleeding at any site can occur as an adverse effect of anticoagulant therapy. If serious bleeding occurs during warfarin therapy, intravenous injection of phytomenadione (vitamin K_1) produces a marked reduction in the prolonged prothrombin time in about 6 h.

The most common indication for anticoagulant therapy is in the treatment of deep vein thrombosis and pulmonary embolism. Heparin is given initially for the first few days, because of its immediate effect, and anticoagulant therapy is then continued with oral warfarin, usually for several months. Long-term anticoagulant therapy is given to those with increased risk of thromboembolism, e.g. patients with mitral valve disease and atrial fibrillation. Prophylactic therapy, using subcutaneous heparin injections, is being used in an attempt to prevent venous thrombosis during periods of recumbency, as following myocardial infarction or peri-and post-operatively.

Any bleeding tendency is a contraindication to anticoagulant therapy. Peptic ulceration, severe hypertension and bacterial endocarditis are also usually regarded as contraindications. Significant hepatic or renal functional impairment is a relative contraindication, as the safe control of dosage may be difficult.

Warfarin shows interactions with several other drugs. Thus, the anticoagulant effect may be increased by the concurrent administration of aspirin or indomethacin and decreased by barbiturates, phenytoin or chlorpromazine. It is essential that the safety of the warfarin dosage is checked by measurement of the prothrombin time or thrombotest whenever any change is made in other drug therapy which the patient is receiving.

If emergency surgery is required for a patient on warfarin therapy, intravenous phytomenadione should be given. However, for less urgent surgical procedures and for dental extraction, it is usually sufficient to omit warfarin therapy for two days prior to the operation.

The prothrombin time or thrombotest must be checked before operating. In patients on long-term anticoagulation, the danger of stopping warfarin has to be balanced against the danger of haemorrhage during surgery and the case should be managed in collaboration with the physician.

7 Leukaemia, lymphadenopathy and lymphoma

Leukaemia

The various types of leukaemia are malignant diseases in which abnormally proliferating cells of the leucocyte series infiltrate the bone marrow and other tissue. Usually the abnormal leucocytes appear in the peripheral blood. In the bone marrow, the malignant cells replace the normal cells so that severe impairment of haematopoiesis may result, causing anaemia, lack of normal granulocytes with increased susceptibility to infections, and thrombocytopenia, leading to a haemorrhagic tendency.

Acute leukaemias

In acute leukaemia there is a great increase in primitive (blast) cells in the marrow which can usually be seen in the blood. In childhood, the leukaemia is usually *lymphoblastic* in type, whereas in adults, it more commonly involves the primitive cells of the granulocyte series— *myeloblastic*.

In acute leukaemia, anaemia may be severe, and haemorrhage and infections are major recurrent problems. Infections of the mouth and throat are common; there may be extensive infection of the gums, with ulceration and bleeding. Sometimes gingival hypertrophy occurs from infiltration with leukaemic cells. Lymph node enlargement occurs, especially in the lymphoblastic type.

Treatment of acute leukaemia is by repeated courses of *multiple cytotoxic drug therapy*, *transfusions* of red cells or platelets as required and intensive *antibiotic treatment* of infections. Without treatment, acute leukaemia is rapidly fatal. In acute lymphoblastic leukaemia in children, considerable success has been achieved with modern cytotoxic therapy. In about 90% of patients, remission can be obtained, with disappearance of all evidence of disease. Although relapses occur, over 40% are still well after five years and many of these can probably be regarded as cured. In acute myeloblastic leukaemia in adults the results of cytotoxic therapy have not been so good. About 70% of patients obtain remission during therapy, but almost all relapse within three years. The development of *bone marrow transplantation* has brought new hope to the management of this type of leukaemia. Although there are many problems and complications associated with marrow transplant, it seems that at least some patients may achieve prolonged survival or even cure.

Chronic myeloid leukaemia

This type of leukaemia occurs mainly in middle life. The main clinical features are those of anaemia, with enlargement of the spleen which may become enormous. There may be weight loss, night sweats and general malaise; sometimes there is a haemorrhagic tendency. Examination of the blood shows anaemia and a greatly elevated leucocyte count, most of the cells being of the granulocyte series. The average duration of life, once diagnosis is made, is about four years. However, there is a large individual variation, and some patients survive for 10 years or more. In most cases, the disease ultimately converts into an *acute blast-cell leukaemia* which is then rapidly fatal. No form of present-day therapy appears to influence the ultimate development of a fatal acute leukaemia. However, in most cases it is possible to keep the patient in reasonably good health during the period of the chronic phase with the cytotoxic drug busulphan.

Chronic lymphatic leukaemia

This disease occurs mainly in the middle and later years of life. The clinical features are progressive enlargement of lymph nodes and spleen, anaemia, sometimes thrombocytopenia, and increased susceptibility to infections. The leucocyte count in the peripheral blood is increased, most of the cells being mature lymphocytes.

The disease varies very much in its rate of progression. Some elderly patients require no treatment over several years as the disease develops very slowly. Treatment is not curative but only palliative, so that it should not be started until the manifestations of the disease warrant interference. Where there is widespread enlargement of lymph nodes, or marrow infiltration with resulting anaemia, treatment is with the cytotoxic drug chlorambucil. For massive enlargement of one group of lymph nodes or of the spleen radiotherapy may be used. The development of autoimmune haemolytic anaemia or thrombocytopenia is fairly common. It is important to distinguish these from the effects of marrow infiltration, as the treatment of the autoimmune complication is with prednisolone.

Myeloma

Myeloma is a malignant proliferation of plasma cells which infiltrate the bone marrow and other tissues. The abnormal plasma cells produce a paraprotein—an abnormal immunoglobulin which can be identified by electrophoresis of plasma. The normal immunoglobulins are reduced, with impaired defence against infections. The amount of abnormal protein may be great enough to increase the viscosity of blood so much as to cause clinical effects. The serum calcium is often raised, anaemia occurs and renal failure is a common complication. The myeloma tumour developing in the marrow may cause erosion of bone with local pain, X-ray appearances of an osteolytic lesion and even pathological fracture. The diagnosis is made from the triad of osteolytic lesions of bone, malignant plasma cell infiltration of the marrow and abnormal protein on plasma electrophoresis. Treatment is by the cytotoxic drug melphalan, usually in combination with other cytotoxics and local radiotherapy for painful bony lesions.

Lymphadenopathy and lymphoma

The lymph nodes are involved in a large variety of disease processes. In many of these, the effect of the disease is to cause an enlargement of the lymph nodes which may then become easily palpable. In some diseases, the enlarged lymph nodes may become enormous.

Lymph node enlargement may be generalized, involving most, or all, of the lymph node areas of the body, or it may be localized, affecting one area only. This is of considerable diagnostic signficance, as a generalized lymphadenopathy indicates a general systemic disease whereas a localized group of enlarged nodes suggests that they have become involved in infection or malignancy in the area from which the nodes are draining lymph. However, sometimes no absolute distinction can be made clinically, as what appears to be a localized group of enlarged nodes is part of a generalized disease, the rest of which is not apparent on clinical examination. Direct palpation can reveal enlarged nodes in the cervical, axillary and inguinal regions. Enlarged intrathoracic nodes in the mediastinum and intra-abdominal nodes in the para-aortic, mesenteric and iliac areas cannot be palpated except at operation and require special radiological techniques for their identification.

The main categories of conditions causing *lymph node enlargement* are as follows:
1. *Infections*
   Bacterial: acute, e.g. streptococcal, staphylococcal,
   Bacterial: chronic, e.g. tuberculosis,
   Viral, e.g. infectious mononucleosis.
2. *Neoplastic*
   Lymphoma, lymphocytic leukaemia,
   Carcinoma.
3. *Auto-immune disease*
   e.g. systemic lupus erythematosus.
4. *Sarcoidosis*
   A granulomatous disorder of unknown aetiology.

Certain characteristics of enlarged lymph nodes are of diagnostic significance. Lymph nodes involved in lymphoma are usually firm, rubbery, discrete, moveable but not tender. Secondary carcinoma causes enlarged nodes which are very hard and fixed to surrounding tissues. In acute infections, the enlarged nodes are tender and the overlying skin may be warm and erythematous. In chronic infections, nodes are usually not tender and may be matted together.

Lymphoma

The lymphomas are a group of malignant diseases of the lymphoid system. Malignant lymphomas can be divided, on the basis of the histological appearances, into two main groups—*Hodgkin's disease* and *non-Hodgkin's lymphoma*. Each of these is further subdivided, according to histological type of tumour, into several subtypes with differing significance for prognosis and response to treatment. Biopsy of an enlarged lymph node or other accessible tumour is essential in making the diagnosis of lymphoma and in determining the precise histological type.

The clinical features of the various malignant lymphomas are similar and include enlargement of lymph nodes and spleen, involvement of the bone marrow with functional impairment and extranodal lymphomatous tumours in liver, lungs, skin and bones. In addition there may be fatigue, intermittent fever, night sweats and weight loss. Painless enlargement of lymph nodes in the neck is a common presentation of Hodgkin's disease; lymphomatous involvement of the tonsil is more likely to be non-Hodgkin's in type. However, the precise type of lymphoma cannot be determined with certainty from clinical examination and biopsy with microscopical examination is necessary.

The prognosis and optimum treatment depend not only on the histological type but also on the extent, or stage of the disease. As well as clinical examination, a range of radiological and scanning techniques are used to determine the extent of involvement of the lymphoma.

The treatment of malignant lymphoma is by radiotherapy for localized disease, and by multiple cytotoxic drug chemotherapy where there is more extensive malignant involvement. The prognosis has improved dramatically following the use of modern radiotherapy and chemotherapy. Of patients with localized Hodgkin's disease treated by radiotherapy, 80–90% are well and free from evidence of disease after five years; many of these can be regarded as cured. When cytotoxic chemotherapy is given for more extensive disease, about 50% of patients have five year disease-free survival. In non-Hodgkin's lymphoma, the prognosis is more variable. Some types of lymphoma progress very slowly over many years, whereas others behave as much more aggressive malignant tumours. Nevertheless, prolonged remissions can be obtained in many patients with radiotherapy or cytotoxic chemotherapy separately or in combination.

8   Principles of management of malignant disease

Malignant disease may be treated by surgery, radiotherapy, cytotoxic drugs or endocrine therapy. Treatment is more likely to be successful when the diagnosis is made early, before local or distant spread of the neoplasm has occurred.

There are many different forms of malignant disease, with different behaviour and clinical presentation. Not every lump is due to neoplasm. Spread to involve local structures and painless involvement of local lymph nodes are features which suggest malignancy. *Biopsy* is necessary to confirm the diagnosis of malignant disease and to determine the histological type of the tumour. Treatment and prognosis vary greatly depending on the precise nature of the tumour.

Once the histological diagnosis has been established, it is then necessary to determine the extent of the disease (its stage) as this may have a major influence on the plan of treatment. An example is the staging scheme for malignant lymphoma, a neoplastic disease of lymphoid cells giving rise to solid tissue tumours:

Stage I: Local involvement of lymph nodes in one region.

Stage II: Lymph node involvement of two or more regions on the same side of the diaphragm.

Stage III: Lymph node involvement both above and below the diaphragm.

Stage IV: Disseminated disease with involvement of extranodal sites, e.g. bone, lung, liver.

This stage of malignant disease is usually arrived at by combining information obtained by: (1) clinical examination and (2) special investigations such as chest radiograph and isotope liver scan and histopathological examination of excised tissue. In general, the higher the stage the poorer is the prognosis.

Surgical treatment
Prophylactic. For example, the removal of the colon in longstanding ulcerative colitis, to prevent subsequent malignant change.

Radical. Excision of localized growths, together with their lymph nodes. The latter should always be examined histologically in order to determine if spread has occurred, e.g. in carcinoma of the breast, a mastectomy is performed together with removal of axillary lymph nodes. Where there is involvement of adjacent structures, e.g. the pectoral muscles in some cases of breast cancer, these may have to be removed. Radiotherapy may also be used in addition to surgery.

Palliative. Where there is an extensive malignant lesion or widespread metastases, local removal of the tumour will not be curative. Surgery, often with radiotherapy or chemotherapy, sometimes has a place in treatment of a troublesome local ulcer or in the symptomatic relief of an inconveniently large mass.

Radiotherapy
The biological effect of radiation is greater in actively dividing cells than in cells in the resting phase. Malignant tumours, which often have a high cell turnover, are therefore sensitive to radiation. Unfortunately, so are some normal cell systems such as the bone marrow stem cells and the intestinal mucosa. Normal tissues, however, recover more quickly from radiation damage to cell enzymes and chromosomal DNA and it is largely this differential recovery rate which makes possible the treatment of cancer by radiotherapy.

The biological effect of radiation on cells is dependent on three factors: the dose of radiation given; the time over which it is administered; and the stage of cell division at the time of exposure.

Radiation may be produced by radioactive substances such as radium or caesium, or from X-ray machines. Radioactive substances may emit three types of radiation:
1. *Alpha particles*: these are very weak and non-penetrating and are of no medical value.
2. *Beta particles (or electrons)*: these are of medium penetration giving intense irradiation over a few millimetres and are mainly used for superficial skin and eye lesions.
3. *Gamma rays*: these are powerfully penetrating and the most useful in the treatment of cancer. Needles or tubes containing a gamma emitting isotope such as caesium may be implanted in tumours (as in carcinoma of the tongue) or inserted in the body cavities (as in carcinoma of the uterine body or cervix).

The majority of patients are, however, treated by X-ray therapy of which there are also three types:

(a) *Superficial X-ray therapy*: a weakly penetrating beam used for the treatment of skin cancer.

(b) *Conventional or 'deep' X-rays*: these are moderately penetrating and are used to treat lesions comparatively near the body surface, such as bone metastases.

(c) *Supervoltage or 'megavoltage' X-rays*: very penetrating well-defined beams used to treat deep-seated tumours. Often several beams are directed to the tumour from different angles thus increasing the dose to the tumour while keeping irradiation of normal tissue to a minimum.

Radiation may be used 'radically', that is, with intent to cure, where it can be highly successful in localized disease such as early carcinoma of the larynx or localized lymphomas. It may also be used palliatively to relieve symptoms in incurable patients and is of particular value in controlling pain due to bone marrow metastases.

Radiotherapy is, of course, not without side effects. If large volumes are irradiated the symptoms tend to be general such as tiredness and nausea, and the peripheral blood picture must be monitored since bone marrow depression may occur. With localized treatment there is transient itch and erythema of the treated skin or inflammation of mucous membranes. With carefully planned and administered radiotherapy, however, severe, acute or long-term morbidity is uncommon.

Cytotoxic drug therapy

Cytotoxic drugs impair cell division by interfering with the synthesis of DNA, RNA or protein. An ideal antineoplastic drug would act only upon tumour cells. However, at present this ideal has not been reached and all cytotoxic drugs which are effective against malignant cells also have some action on normal cells. As the effect is greatest on those cells dividing most rapidly, the normal tissues most likely to be damaged include the bone marrow and the epithelium of the alimentary tract.

A given dose of a cytotoxic drug kills a constant fraction of cells, regardless of the total number of cells present. Because of this, when there are a large number of malignant cells present, as in advanced disease, it may not be possible to eradicate the neoplasm, because the dose of cytotoxic drug required would be greater than could be tolerated by the normal cells. In early disease, where there is only a relatively small number of malignant cells, complete eradication may be possible.

Tumours vary greatly in their response to cytotoxic drugs. With a few types of malignancy, for example Hodgkin's disease, acute lymphoblastic leukaemia in childhood and choriocarcinoma, cure is possible. With others, e.g. non-Hodgkin's lymphoma, myeloma, chronic myeloid leukaemia, while cure may not be possible, prolonged control of the disease may be achieved. Some tumours, for example gastrointestinal carcinoma and squamous bronchial carcinoma, usually show little response to presently available chemotherapy.

Combinations of cytotoxic drugs are frequently used, giving several drugs which have different biochemical actions on the cell, which attack the cell at different phases of the growth cycle, and which may have differing toxicities. Commonly, intermittent chemotherapy is used, allowing intervals for recovery of the normal cells between periods of chemotherapy.

The following normal tissues may be adversely affected by cytotoxic chemotherapy:

1. *Bone marrow.* Anaemia, leucopenia (causing increased susceptibility to infections) and thrombocytopenia (leading to the danger of haemorrhage).
2. *Lymphoid system.* Immunosuppression—increasing susceptibility to and severity of infections.
3. *Mucosa of alimentary tract.* Diarrhoea, ulceration of the mouth.
4. *Hair follicles.* Loss of hair.
5. *Gonadal cells.* May cause sterility. Because of possibility of mutagenicity, pregnancy should be avoided curing cytotoxic therapy.
6. *Delayed wound healing.*

In addition to these general effects of cytotoxic drugs, some such drugs have specific toxicities, e.g. pulmonary fibrosis with bleomycin and cardiomyopathy with doxorubicin.

Cytotoxic drugs interfere with the metabolism of dividing cells in one of several ways:

(a) *Alkylating agents—damage to DNA*, e.g. cyclophosphamide, busulphan.
(b) *Interference with purine metabolism*, e.g. mercaptopurine, azathioprine.
(c) *Interference with pyrimidine metabolism*, e.g. fluorouracil, cytarabine.
(d) *Folic acid antagonism*, e.g. methotrexate.

(e) *Plant alkaloids which cause cell arrest in mitosis*, e.g. vincristine, vinblastine.
(f) *Antibiotics which interfere with DNA synthesis*, e.g. doxorubicin, bleomycin.

Endocrine therapy

Some types of malignant disease are hormone-sensitive and the use of sex hormones or hormone antagonists may inhibit their growth. Tamoxifen, an oestrogen antagonist, is used in post-menopausal metastatic breast cancer. Oestrogens, e.g. stilboestrol, are used in prostatic cancer which is androgen-dependent.

9 Immunity, immune deficiency, hypersensitivity and immunization

Immunity, hypersensitivity and immune deficiency are all interelated, the relationship being as represent in Fig. 8.

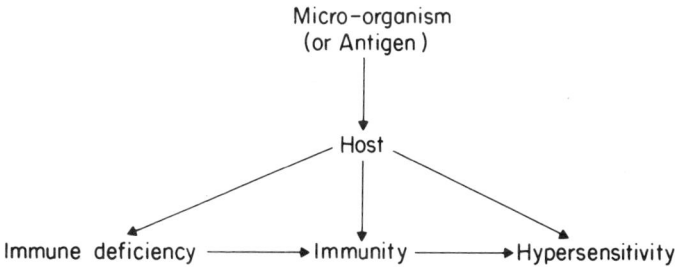

Fig. 8   Immunity, hypersensitivity, and immune deficiency.

Immunity is where the host defence mechanisms respond to an invading organism or antigen, countering its effect by a response which causes no harm to the body.

Immune deficiencies occur when the immune response is less than that required for immunity.

Hypersensitivity occurs when the immune system over-responds and produces a damaging reaction.

Clearly, a new response begins as a deficient response, achieves immunity with the passage of time and does not normally continue into an over-response phase.

Immune mechanisms
These can be divided into:

Innate mechanisms of immunity such as:
1. 'Barrier' effect of skin and mucosae.
2. Protective effect of the commensal micro-organisms of the body.
3. Continuous flow of secretions (saliva, mucus and intestinal contents).
4. Limitation of nutrient material (e.g. skin).
5. Protective effect of antimicrobial substances:
   Fatty acids in skin,
   Lysozyme in tears and other secretions,
   Interferon: protein which inhibits viral replication.

Effector mechanisms of immunity such as phagocytic cells in the body. The most important are:
1. *Polymorphonuclear leucocytes (neutrophil type)* which are short-lived cells, produced in large numbers in the blood, which ingest and destroy foreign materials, including bacteria. These cells 'home' in on their targets by responding to specific 'chemotactic signals'.
2. *Macrophages (the tissue forms of monocytes)* are long-lived cells capable of continuing an active phagocytic role for long periods. These cells 'wander' through the tissues locating and ingesting foreign material, and also respond to 'chemotactic signals'.
Both types of cell can be made more efficient in phagocytosis by the provision of a complement factor (C_3b) and IgG antibody. This is called *opsonization* and it is a very important part of the host response to infection.

Macrophages, additionally, have an important role in the presentation of antigens to B-lymphocytes (*see* below), and they can be *directed* to certain activities by T-lymphocytes.

Complement. This is a complex series of nine major proteins which activate in a cascade sequence when triggered by immune complexes (combinations of antigen and antibody). The proteins are numbered from C1 to C9 and the sequence of activation is C1–C2–C4–C3–C5–C6–C7–C8–C9. C9 is lytic to cells and micro-organisms. The breakdown fragment of C3 termed C3b has opsonizing ability (*see* 2 above) and the fragments C3a and C5a are chemotaxins.

Antibody. Antibodies are special proteins produced by plasma cells which specifically bind to foreign substances (antigens). Each antibody formed is specific for a single antigen. Antibodies are found in many body fluids and can be classified in molecular terms into classes of immunoglobulin (IgM, IgG, IgA, IgD and IgE). The different classes have different biological features. Plasma cells themselves are derived from specialized lymphocytes called B-cells (for B-lymphocytes).

After combination of antigen and antibody a variety of biological events may be stimulated, e.g. agglutination of particles, precipitation of soluble antigen, neutralization of toxins or viruses, activation of the complement sequence. A particularly important action of IgG antibody is opsonization.

Cellular immunity. Cellular immunity is effected by T-lymphocytes (T-cells). Each T-cell, or clone of T-cells, reacts specifically with a single antigen. If the antigen is associated with a micro-organism the T-cell activates macrophages to ingest and destroy the organism. This is an important mechanism for removing microbes which produce chronic infections, e.g. Brucella, Mycobacteria, Candida, Leishmania, and which are usually unaffected by neutrophils, complement and antibody.

T-cells also produce a direct cytolytic effect, which is important in the response to intracellular parasites such as viruses. In such an instance, the cell, with its contained viruses, is destroyed, and the T-cells involved are called T-effector lymphocytes.

There are other types of T-cells which are involved in the control of antibody and T-effector activities. These are helper T-cells which potentiate the response and suppressor T-cells which decrease the response. Memory T-cells retain the ability to respond quickly to a given antigen.

Cellular immunity is particularly involved in defence against certain categories of parasite (*see* above), in transplanted graft rejections and in the control of tumours.

Integration of the response

It is important to remember that the response to foreign materials and/or micro-organisms is usually integrated. Thus the effect of polymorphs, macrophages, complement, antibody and T-cells are combined to produce immunity. Where one or more of these components is underactive an immune deficiency results; where they are overactive hypersensitivity occurs.

Immune deficiency
Immune deficiencies can be divided into two broad categories:
1. Those which are inherited and are associated with absence of a
   particular cell or protein. These are rare.
2. Those in which the immune system is intact but where it fails to
   respond adequately to a challenge.

Inherited (congenital)
1. Inherited defects of polymorphonuclear leucocytes and macrophages occur where the cells have no ability to kill micro-organisms.
   The best known example is chronic granulomatous disease which
   is associated with chronic bacterial infections of skin and mucous
   membranes.
2. Absence of several of the complement components has been
   described. Often these deficiencies are not associated with clinical
   abnormalities, but in some instances, such as C7 deficiency, frequent, serious bacterial infections, e.g. meningococcal meningitis,
   occur.
3. Defects of B-lymphocytes result in failure to produce antibody,
   the clinical condition being termed hypogammaglobulinaemia. The
   most extreme form is called Bruton's disease where there is vir-
   tually no antibody present in serum. This condition is associated
   with severe bacterial infections (pneumonias, meningitis, etc.) and
   death occurs early in life in untreated patients.
       Lesser degrees of hypogammaglobulinaemia occur, where
   there is reduction in the amount of IgG, or IgA, or IgM. These
   deficiencies may be associated with a higher incidence of bacterial
   infection, although many patients appear to be normal.
4. T-cell deficiencies lead to defects of immunity to viruses. The
   commonest representative is *Di George syndrome* (*thymic aplasia*)
   in which otherwise trivial viral infections such as chickenpox and
   measles become life-threatening. Immunity to tumour formation
   is also decreased in these patients.
5. When T-cell and B-cell deficiencies coexist the condition is referred
   to as severe combined immune deficiency syndrome (Swiss type).
   In its most severe form it is incompatible with survival and death
   from serious viral or bacterial infections occurs within a few months
   of birth.
6. AIDS—or acquired immune deficiency syndrome is a topical,
   though rare disease. It is characterized by profound depression
   of T-cell immunity, associated with increased numbers of

T-suppressor cells and decreased numbers of T-helper cells. Clinically, problems arise. because these patients have a high incidence of tumours (particularly Kaposi's sarcoma) and an increased susceptibility to otherwise harmless organisms such as *Pneumocystis carinii*. It is thought to be caused by HTLV3 virus which is transmitted sexually or by blood transfusion or inoculation.

Functional immune deficiencies

These are sometimes produced by interference (i.e. drug or other treatment) but on other occasions they appear to be spontaneous and probably represent milder versions of the rare conditions described above in inherited (congenital) defects.

It should be clear from the discussion earlier that any immune response which is less efficient than that which produces immunity is an immune deficiency. In this respect *all* infections are examples of immune deficiency and it is important to examine for all aspects of immune dysfunction and correct deficiencies where possible, in order to provide the best care for the patient. An example which illustrates this is candidosis, an infection due to *Candida albicans*.

C. albicans is an inhabitant of the commensal flora of all healthy persons, being found chiefly in the mouth and intestinal tract. The number of organisms present in these sites varies from person to person but is constant over long periods in any individual. There is continuous production of antibody which can be found in serum and secretions and cellular immunity is also highly developed. There is a balance, in the normal person, between the population of the organism in the body and the response which is mounted against it, and infection *only* occurs when this balance is disrupted. The factors which are known to disturb the balance are briefly as follows:

1. Mechanical damage to mucosal barriers (innate immunity) as caused by badly fitting dentures. Correction of the mechanical problem cures the patient and antifungal therapy is unnecessary.
2. Iron and folate deficiency produces mucosal defects which predipose to infection in the mouth and vagina. Replacement therapy corrects the defect and cures the patient.
3. Antibiotic therapy disturbs the normal flora of the intestinal tract. The normal flora constitutes a 'barrier' and loss of this activity allows *C. albicans* to overgrow and produce infection. These infections resolve quickly when the antibiotics are stopped.
4. Systemic candida infections occur when there is a failure to produce sufficient serum antibody to cope with a large increase in local

growth of the organism. Spillover of the organism into the blood occurs with seeding of other tissues and organs. This event often follows the administration of cytotoxic drugs (for cancer treatment) which suppress antibody formation.

5. Deficiency of T-cell activity against *C. albicans* occurs in a severe form in the rare inherited condition *chronic mucocutaneous candidosis*, and in a milder form in many women with chronic candida infections of the vagina, mouth, throat and oesophagus. These patients are easily identified by a simple skin test using candida antigen to which they produce no response at all. Correction of this defect may be possible by immunotherapy (transfer factor) or using the drug Inosiplex. Without correction of the immune deficiency, cure is impossible.

   Similar cases are due to treatment with drugs which depress T-cell activity. The most commonly encountered are corticosteroids, but cytotoxic drugs and radiotherapy have the same effect.

6. Women taking oral contraceptives have a higher incidence of candida infections. The mechanism here is not known with certainty but it is established that oestrogens and prostogens modify T-cell immune responsiveness.

From the example above it should be clear that it is no longer acceptable to label a patient 'immunodeficient', or 'immunocompromised' and do nothing to clarify the basic problem. Whenever one sees an infection, particularly a chronic infection, a checklist of possible immunological causes should spring to mind and each should be investigated. As in the case of candidosis, above, different defects of immune activity can produce different clinical presentations and knowledge of these leads to a rational approach to management of the patient. There are, however, some 'golden rules' to be observed in any immunodeficient patient:

(a) Resist the temptation to prescribe a battery of powerful, broad-spectrum antibiotics. These will often 'select out' a very resistant organism which will kill the patient.

(b) Never use *live vaccines* when immunizing a patient with immune deficiency for these may produce fatal infections. This is particularly important in the case of children taking corticosteroids.

(c) Remember that all patients with Hodgkin's lymphoma are severely immunodeficient (T-cells), and many patients with cancer similarly so.

(d) Malnutrition is the commonest cause of immune deficiency in global terms. In the UK, malnutrition exists in certain sectors of the community (particularly the old). Correction of the nutritional problem solves the immune deficiency problem (*see* candidosis, above).

Hypersensitivity

As indicated earlier hypersensitivity has two important characteristics:

1. It is an over-response by some part of the immune system,
2. It produces damage in the body.

Hypersensitivities are clinically classified into four major types according to the Gell and Coombs classification.

Type 1 is called anaphylactic hypersensitivity and is due to antibody of the IgE class. This antibody attaches to mast cells and sensitizes them such that further contact with the stimulating antigen triggers the mast cells to release histamine. The main clinical effects of histamine release are vasodilatation and bronchoconstriction. If the release of histamine is small and locally contained, the clinical effects are mild. On the other hand, massive, systemic release of histamine can lead to death within a few minutes by causing shock and breathing difficulties. The latter condition is termed *generalized anaphylaxis*.

Normal people produce only small amounts of IgE antibody when responding to new antigens, but 10% of the population fail to control the production of IgE, over-respond and become susceptible to anaphylactic reactions. These people are termed 'atopic'.

Type 2 hypersensitivity occurs when antibody is produced against antigens on the surface of one's own cells. The antibody attaches to the cells, activates complement and the cells may be destroyed or severely damaged. This reaction is one of the bases of *autoimmune* disease, and is manifest in diseases such as acquired haemolytic anaemia. Clearly, the inability to control the antibody response to self-antigens represents an over-response of the immune system.

A variant of this mechanism occurs where 'haptens' (molecules which themselves are not antigenic) attach to cell surfaces and become antigenic. The antibody which is produced against the haptens attaches and activates complement and the cell is destroyed. Drugs are important haptens in this respect and may induce haemolytic anaemias, thrombocytopenic purpura or, in the case of antibiotics, neutropenia.

Chapter 9

Type 3 hypersensitivity is due to the formation in the body of excess quantities of immune complexes. The latter are formed by combination of soluble antigen and antibody (usually IgG) and at certain ratios (of antigen/antibody) they activate complement. If the complexes are in the tissues, the complement activation attracts neutrophils which then damage the tissues. The amount of damage resulting is dependent on how much complex forms and for how long it persists. The distribution of the lesions largely depends on whether the complexes form locally, e.g. in skin, lung, or systemically. In the latter instance the kidneys are particularly likely to be damaged because the high blood flow carries the complexes into the glomeruli and glomerulonephritis results. Other important organs and tissues are also damaged, e.g. joints, muscles and peripheral blood vessels.

Immune complex damage plays an important part in rheumatic fever, in the systemic effects of infective endocarditis, rheumatoid arthritis, systemic lupus erythematosus and serum sickness.

Type 4 hypersensitivity is a manifestation of an over-active T-cell response. A classical, but not isolated example is seen in tuberculosis. Effective removal or control of the tubercle bacilli requires T-cell sensitization and the involvement of macrophages. If the T-cells are over-reactive, macrophages damage the tissues, rather than restricting their activity to the micro-organisms. Much of the lung damage in tuberculosis is due to this type of hypersensitivity.

General comments
It is always tempting to think of hypersensitivity reactions as being one or other of the above mechanisms, but it is worth remembering that a single antigen can induce one or more of the types of response described. A good example is penicillin which is known to induce Type 1, Type 3 and Type 4 reactions. Type 1 hypersensitivity due to penicillin is the rarest form, although potentially the most serious because it can induce generalized anaphylaxis. Many patients who state that they are 'penicillin allergic' have had mild Type 3 or Type 4 reactions in the past and would be inconvenienced if given the drug again. However, penicillins are usually excluded for all patients with a history of reaction in order to avoid the rare chance of a Type 1 reaction.

Local anaesthesia preparations also induce hypersensitivities which can be of Type 1 variety. When assessing the risk of a reaction in an individual it is common practice to enquire as to general allergy, e.g. to foods, fish, proteins, etc. The reason is simply that 'atopic' patients are predisposed to Type 1 reactions which can be induced by many antigens including drugs and therefore care should be taken when treating these patients.

Immunization

Immunization is the procedure by which one induces immunity in the host to micro-organisms, using vaccines which contain the organisms in a safe, but antigenic form. The induction of immunity is a complex process but some general points are worthy of note:

1. Vaccines which contain killed organisms, e.g. typhoid and pertussis vaccines, are generally poor inducers of immune responses. This is probably because the antigenic challenge is 'short and sharp' and quite unlike the progressive build-up of organisms one sees in a 'wild' infection. Consequently, several doses of such vaccines have to be given and booster injections may be required to maintain immunity. Even then immunity is only induced in a proportion of individuals. The aim is to protect as many as possible and usually these vaccines will induce immunity in 60–80% of persons. However, because of the variability of immune responses in the population, some persons will remain unprotected even if properly immunized. These individuals may have partial protection, or none.

2. *Adjuvants* are substances which increase immune responsiveness. Some, such as mineral oils and *Mycobacterium tuberculosis*, are too powerful for use in routine immunization. *Alum precipitation* is frequently used (as in some tetanus toxoid vaccines) the antigen being adsorbed on to aluminium hydroxide particles. The release of antigen in the body is slow and sustained and mimics the natural disease more closely.

   Bordetella pertussis is itself a powerful adjuvant and when given with tetanus and diptheria toxoids (as in the triple vaccine) boosts the response to the toxoids.

3. Vaccines should in theory enter the body through the same routes as the natural infection in order to induce immunity in the area that matters. Often, vaccines are ineffective because they do not conform to this general rule, e.g. influenza vaccines which are administered intramuscularly, when in fact immunity of the respiratory mucosa is required.

This said, the development of vaccines which mimic the natural infection is difficult.

4. Live, attenuated vaccines, where the organisms have been weakened, are generally much more successful than killed organisms or purified antigens. The reason for this is that the attenuated organisms multiply to a limited extent (never producing disease) in the body and produce a steady increase of antigen in the same way as the wild infection. *Live vaccines must not be administered to immunodeficient individuals.*

Table 2   Schedule of immunization.

Age	Vaccines	Comments
3 or 6 months 5 or 8 months 9 or 12 months	*Triple and oral polio *Triple and oral polio *Triple and oral polio	Diphtheria and tetanus toxoid may be given without the pertussis component. Alum adsorbed vaccines must be used in this case
1 – 2 years	Measles [live]	At least three weeks apart from any other live vaccine
4 – 5 years	Diphtheria/tetanus toxoids and oral polio	
10 – 13 years	BCG—for tuberculosis	Given only to tuberculin-negative children
11 – 13 years (girls only)	Rubella vaccine	
15 – 19 years	Tetanus toxoid and oral polio	Reinforce every 10 years

Triple vaccine contains tetanus toxoid, diphtheria toxoid, *Bordetella pertussis* (killed organisms).

5. Tetanus and diphtheria vaccines, which are toxoids, are highly successful because the amount of antibody which needs to be induced for protection is very small. Hence three doses of these toxoids will induce solid protection.

6. A good example of a successful vaccine is the oral (live) polio vaccine. The vaccine strain is harmless and stable (i.e. does not revert to a virulent form). It induces solid immunity which lasts for

5–10 years and protects the important part of the body, the gut, because of its oral administration.

Immunization requirements vary from country to country depending on local considerations and there is even variance from area to area in the UK. In general, however, the recommendations in the UK are as listed in Table 2.

10 Gastrointestinal disorders

The gastrointestinal, alimentary, or digestive tract comprises the mouth through to the anus, with all the appendages of that system, including the salivary glands, liver, gall-bladder and pancreas.

Anatomical and physiological considerations
Abnormalities of dentition may govern the degree of mastication or even influence the type of food consumed.

During the process of swallowing, food initially passes into the pharynx. At this level swallowing is under voluntary control and powered by striated muscle. Thus lesions of nervous, e.g. bulbar or pseudobulbar palsy (p.177), neuromuscular, e.g. myasthenia gravis (p.177), or muscular origin, e.g. polymyositis (p.177), may cause difficulty in swallowing (dysphagia). Below the level of the cricoid cartilage the action of swallowing takes place in the oesophagus where it is controlled by the autonomic nervous system and powered by smooth muscle. Immediately below the diaphragm the oesophagus opens into the cardia of the stomach at the cardio-oesophageal junction where a sphincter mechanism prevents regurgitation of gastric contents.

The stomach acts as a reservoir in which food is mixed and broken into smaller particles, and gradually passed through the pylorus into the duodenum. The secretory function of the gastric mucosa includes hydrochloric acid, pepsin, and intrinsic factor. Hydrochloric acid reduces bacterial contamination of the small intestine and provides the optimum pH for gastric pepsin which initiates digestion. Intrinsic factor binds to vitamin B_{12} facilitating its absorption in the terminal ileum.

The duodenal contents are mixed with bile containing acids and pancreatic secretions which include digestive enzymes and bicarbonate necessary for digestion. Absorption of small molecular weight particles (peptides, fatty acids, etc.) occurs through the mucosa of the jejunum and ileum. A few substances are preferentially absorbed from specific sites, e.g. iron from the proximal jejunum and vitamin B_{12} from the terminal ileum.

The terminal ileum joins the colon at the caecum where a valve prevents retrograde flow of intestinal contents, and thus contamination of the small intestine by bacteria which may impair absorption. Water and electrolytes are absorbed throughout the colon resulting in a semi-formed stool which is passed from the rectum.

The liver has many important functions. It synthesizes proteins including clotting factors, maintains blood glucose values from stored glycogen, filters both portal and systemic blood, so removing and detoxifying materials such as drugs, and secretes bilirubin (a breakdown product of haemoglobin) and bile acids which play an important role in the absorption of fat and fat-soluble vitamins. The pancreas has exocrine and endocrine functions. The exocrine secretion includes bicarbonate and digestive enzymes which are secreted in response to hormones which are released when food enters the duodenum. The most important endocrine function is insulin production without which the patient develops diabetes.

Oral manifestations of systemic disease
Clues to several general medical disorders are to be found in the face and mouth. For example:

Eyes: Yellow tint with jaundice, e.g. due to haemolysis in pernicious anaemia,

Lips: Blue with cyanosis, due to inadequate oxygenation of blood,

Mouth: Cracked at corners, due to iron deficiency,

Gums: Bleeding easily, due to blood dyscrasias, especially monocytic leukaemia or scurvy (vitamin C deficiency),
Hypertrophied due to prolonged phenytoin therapy (p.182),
Discoloured blue due to lead poisoning (p.169),

Tongue: Furred, e.g. in large bowel neoplasms,
Smooth and sore in deficiencies of iron, vitamin B_1, B_2, B_6, B_{12}, nicotinic acid (niacin) and folic acid,
Large, in patients with myxoedema, acromegaly and amyloidosis,
Small and spastic in motor neurone disease,

Breath: Characteristic odours of breath, such as the sweet smell of ketones in untreated diabetes, the faeculent smell in appendicitis.

Lips
Can be the site of primary tumours, particularly squamous cell carcinoma: most common in pipe smokers.

Mouth

The mucosal lining of the mouth can also undergo malignant change, predisposing factors being leukoplakia, chronic dental ulcer and syphilis. Ulceration can be aphthous, the cause of which is largely unknown, infective—either fungal, syphilitic or tuberculous—or neoplastic, when the base is indurated and the edge rolled and regional lymph nodes may be palpable. Oral candidosis occurs in the debilitated, especially after broad-spectrum antibiotics. A gross form of this, acute pseudomembranous candidosis, occurs in immunosuppressed patients. Painful shallow aphthous-type ulcers often occur in association with coeliac disease and inflammatory bowel disease, particularly Crohn's disease, which very occasionally causes a nodular non-caseating granuloma in the mouth. An extremely rare oral manifestation of ulcerative colitis is pyostomatitis vegetans, the initial lesions of which appear as tiny abscesses on a red base. Later these enlarge and become confluent and may then vegetate. Their course corresponds to the remissions and exacerbations of the colonic disease. The surfaces affected are the gingivae, mucosal surfaces of the lips, and the mucobuccal folds. The oral cavity may be affected by mucocutaneous diseases such as pemphigus and erythema multiforme (Stevens–Johnson syndrome) which may arise as a reaction to sulphonamides or mycoplasma infections.

Xerostomia is the symptom of dry mouth. The commonest cause of this is disorder of the salivary glands. Examples include degeneration after radiotherapy for oral cancer, infiltrating lesions involving the salivary glands, such as leukaemia, lymphoma, sarcoidosis and Waldenstrom's macroglobulinaemia. A dry mouth can be caused by drugs, e.g. anticholinergic agents and certain tranquillizers. The symptom may accompany the excess thirst of uncontrolled diabetes mellitus and chronic renal failure, and is dominant in disorders specific to the salivary glands such as Mikulicz's and Sjörgen's disease (*see* below).

Ptyalism is the symptom of excessive secretion of saliva. It can be caused by:
1. Inflammatory lesions of the mouth,
2. Parkinson's disease,
3. Heavy metal poisoning, e.g. mercury (p.169),
4. Carcinoma of the tongue,
5. Excessive iodide intake,
6. Psychiatric disturbance.

Drooling is the leakage of saliva from the mouth. It is usually associated with paralysis of some of the muscles around the mouth.

Salivary glands

Disorders of these usually present with local swelling, sometimes with pain in addition. Inflammation can be due to organisms such as the mumps virus, pus-forming bacteria, and obstruction, particularly duct stenosis and calculi. Calculi occur most commonly in the submandibular gland, and are found here or in its (Wharton's) duct. Stones in the gland necessitate its removal, whereas those in the duct can usually be removed by an incision into the duct made from within the mouth.

There is a variety of different tumours of salivary glands, the incidence of particular tumours being different in the different glands. The parotid is most frequently affected and can be the site of the benign tumour *adenolymphoma*, the potentially malignant tumour, *pleomorphic adenoma,* and the malignant *carcinoma.* The facial nerve, having an intimate relation with the parotid gland, can be damaged by these growths and by surgery to remove them.

Mikulicz's and *Sjögren's diseases* are classified as autoimmune conditions in which antibodies to salivary gland tissue circulate in the plasma and effectively destroy it. In Mikulicz's disease, which is the rarer, one or all of the salivary glands are enlarged, there is involvement of the lacrimal glands, enlargement of which causes narrowing of the palpebral fissures, and there is intense xerostomia. In Sjögren's disease there is an accompanying polyarthritis similar to rheumatoid arthritis (p.157).

Uveo-parotid fever (Heerfordt's syndrome) due to sarcoidosis (p.68) is characterized by enlargement of the parotid glands, uveitis, and a febrile illness, with malaise. Sometimes this is also accompanied by enlargement of the lacrimal glands and sometimes by facial (7th cranial nerve) palsy.

Pharynx

The hallmarks of pharyngeal diseases are disorders of swallowing, a bodily function of obvious concern to the oral surgeon. Inflammation can be caused by corrosives, bacteria, fungi and viruses and by inappropriate exposure to the normal secretions of the body, such as bile and gastric acid. Difficulty in swallowing, *dysphagia*, can arise from mechanical obstruction:

   Intrinsic, such as web on stricture following prolonged inflammation, or previous surgery, or tumour,

   Extrinsic, such as pouch or aneurysm, neuromuscular lesions such as bulbar palsy and achalasia of the cardia.

Sore throats are usually caused by viral infections. Streptococcal tonsillitis may lead to large inflamed tonsils with beads of pus on their surface. The appearance of a white tonsillar membrane with palatal petechiae is characteristic of glandular fever (infectious mononucleosis, p.288).

Oesophagus

Peptic oesophagitis

Incompetence of the lower oesophageal sphincter permits reflux of gastric contents containing acid, pepsin and sometimes bile acids which damage the oesophageal mucosa causing oesophagitis. The patient complains of a retrosternal burning discomfort (heartburn) when corrosive gastric contents contact the inflamed mucosa. Episodes of heartburn occur after fatty meals which lower the sphincter tone, in association with bending, and at night when the patient is recumbent. Occasionally spasm of the underlying oesophageal muscle provokes severe chest pain of a similar character to that of myocardial infarction.

Peptic oesophagitis is a cause of chronic blood loss and thus of iron deficiency anaemia. Untreated it may lead to fibrosis and narrowing with dysphagia for solid foods which is initially intermittent.

Treatment includes attention to posture, avoiding lying flat, and avoiding any factors known to lower oesophageal sphincter tone such as tobacco, caffeine, excess alcohol and very fatty meals. Antacids give symptomatic relief and alginate-containing preparations such as Gaviscon may provide a protective barrier. H_2-receptor antagonists (cimetidine or ranitidine) are very helpful in some patients, but it must be remembered that alkaline reflux is more corrosive than acid. Metoclopramide increases sphincter tone and gastric emptying; it is useful before retiring. Some patients require surgical procedures to prevent or dilate strictures. Any associated hiatus hernia is repaired at the same time.

Oesophageal carcinoma

This disease is more common in patients who smoke, abuse alcohol, and suffer from coeliac disease. The tumour usually arises in the lower third of the oesophagus and presents with dysphagia for solids. In contrast to peptic stricture, there may be no preceding history of heartburn and the dysphagia is usually progressive until eventually the patient has difficulty in swallowing liquids, even saliva. Malnutrition and weight loss occur early. Where possible the tumour is treated by local excision. Frequently mediastinal or metastatic spread precludes such attempts at curative surgery. Under these circumstances the insertion of a plastic tube into the oesophageal lumen palliates symptoms.

Achalasia of the oesophagus

Neuromuscular incoordination is responsible for the failure of the sphincter to relax, the proximal oesophagus is frequently inert and dilates, and may fill with food debris. The patient complains of dysphagia. Most difficulty is encountered with liquids. Aspiration pneumonia and a propensity to oesophageal carcinoma are other features of this disease. Incision of the muscle at the cardia (cardiomyotomy) relieves the obstruction.

Oesophageal investigations

A barium swallow and meal examination is readily available and provides information about motility and strictures. Endoscopic examination allows direct inspection and biopsy. Oesophageal manometry is required to investigate patients with suspected achalasia.

Stomach and duodenum

When the upper regions of the stomach are above instead of below the diaphragm, the condition is called *hiatus hernia*. There are two types: sliding, associated with reflux of gastric juice into the oesophagus, and rolling, where the herniated part of the stomach is its fundus, which is liable to incarceration.

Peptic ulceration

The term peptic ulceration refers to chronic ulcers which usually occur in the duodenum or stomach. The cause of peptic ulcer disease is uncertain, but the formation of ulcers reflects an imbalance between acid secretion and mucosal protective factors. Small superficial ulcers (erosions) may be caused by drug ingestion, especially non-steroidal anti-inflammatory analgesics; they produce similar symptoms but they are transient.

The symptoms of duodenal ulcers are clinically indistinguishable from those of gastric ulcer disease. Episodic epigastric pain occurs after meals, sometimes wakes the patient at night, and is temporarily relieved by alkalis. However, patients with peptic ulcers may be entirely asymptomatic.

Complications include bleeding, perforation (with peritonitis) and pyloric stenosis. Bleeding may be acute, presenting with vomiting blood (haematemesis) and/or passing tarry motions (melaena), with or without shock, or chronic, resulting in iron deficiency and anaemia. Perforation is heralded by the sudden onset of severe abdominal pain, the abdomen feels hard and tender, and plain X-ray may demonstrate free gas under the diaphragm. Fibrosis induced by an ulcer near the pylorus can cause pyloric stenosis, the patient vomits copiously and eventually complete gastric outlet obstruction occurs. There is a little evidence that gastric ulcers undergo malignant transformation, although it is possible that some such ulcers are malignant from the start.

The aim of treatment is to heal ulcers, prevent complications, and alleviate symptoms. Ulcers may be healed by drugs which suppress acid secretion (cimetidine or ranitidine which are *histamine receptor* H_2-blocking drugs) or drugs which act topically such as bismuth chelate or sucralfate. Only maintenance treatment with H_2-receptor blocking drugs has been shown to reduce the tendency to frequent relapse which occurs in some patients. These two drugs are similar but the use of ranitidine avoids drug interaction and other side effects occasionally caused by cimetidine. Rarely patients require surgery either for intractable ulcers or for complications. Vagotomy and drainage procedure is most commonly employed, but 10% of patients suffer post-gastric surgery complications, the most common being diarrhoea.

Gastric cancer
This tumour presents insidiously with anorexia, epigastric discomfort and weight loss. Proximal and distal tumours may cause obstruction or vomiting. Metastasis to the liver occurs early. Surgery is the only effective treatment. In a few patients curative gastrectomy may be attempted, but frequently only palliative by-pass procedures are possible on account of metastases. Most patients are dead within five years.

Gastritis

Acute gastritis follows the ingestion of excess alcohol; chronic gastritis is associated with bile reflux after surgery; both may cause epigastric pain which is aggravated by food. Chronic atrophic gastritis usually produces no gastric symptoms. It is an autoimmune disorder related to thyroid disease and type I diabetes, and associated with the development of auto-antibodies to gastric mucosa. The most important feature of this disease is the failure to produce intrinsic factor and thus absorb vitamin B_{12} with the eventual development of megaloblastic anaemia (pernicious anaemia). These patients do not secrete gastric acid.

Investigation of the stomach

A barium meal is the traditional method of examining the stomach. It is safe and widely available. Flexible fibre-optic endoscopes which offer direct visualization and biopsy of lesions in the oesophagus, stomach or duodenum are now used increasingly, usually under mild sedation. Gastric acid secretion can be measured, hypersecretion being identified thereby. Some endocrine disorders are associated with high gastric acidity and severe ulceration. These can be diagnosed by serum assay.

Gall-bladder and pancreas

The gall-bladder can be the site of origin of several types of stones (*cholelithiasis*) formed from cholesterol or bile pigments which can give rise to colic, infection and obstruction of either the biliary tree (*cholangitis* and *obstructive jaundice*) or more distal parts of the alimentary tract. Inflammation of the gall-bladder (*cholecystitis*) is usually a sequel to cholelithiasis but may be of the 'acalculous' type, that is without stones being present. Cholecystitis, characterized by upper abdominal pain and vomiting, may settle on treatment with antibiotics, but may go on to an abscess of the gall-bladder, an *empyema*, which has to be drained. Gall-bladder disease is associated with pancreatic disorders, especially *acute pancreatitis*.

Acute pancreatitis presents with severe upper abdominal pain, usually radiating through to the back, and physical signs of peritonitis. Hypocalcaemia and hyperglycaemia can occur too. It is a serious condition in which renal and respiratory failure may cause death. It can be caused by other factors including ingestion of alcohol, certain drugs and viral diseases, particularly mumps and Coxsackie. Cancer of the pancreas is becoming increasingly common. Unfortunately it usually presents too late for radical surgery to cure it and sympto-matic treatment is all that is possible.

Small and large bowel

Diseases of the small bowel are uncommon. They include inherited conditions such as coeliac disease, (in which malabsorption occurs due to hypersensitivity to dietary gluten) and small bowel polyposis (in which about 2% ultimately undergo malignant change). Carcinoid, hormone-secreting tumours may arise from the small bowel, often causing symptoms such as flushing and diarrhoea from the ectopic secretion of serotonin.

The distal small bowel, the terminal ileum, is the commonest site in the alimentary tract for Crohn's disease to occur. This inflammatory bowel disease of unknown aetiology frequently has a chronic course, with acute exacerbations. It causes diarrhoea, malabsorption, weight loss and can be the cause of acute surgical emergencies such as intestinal obstruction and peritonitis. Its management usually requires a combination of medical and surgical treatment.

The caecum, where the small bowel joins the large, is the site of the appendix, that tiny organ which is regarded as vestigial in humans and yet in the west is the commonest cause of emergency surgery. Acute appendicitis has a characteristic history, starting with intermit-tent (so called 'colicky') central abdominal pain, which then moves into the right lower quadrant of the abdomen, the iliac fossa, which becomes increasingly tender to palpation and where peritonitis can begin if appendicectomy is not performed promptly. Vomiting and fever usually accompany the illness and diarrhoea can occur. The breath is usually foul smelling and the tongue coated grey-brown. As long as the diagnosis is made early on in the illness, appendicectomy can usually be performed simply, and rapid, uneventful recovery be expected. Acute appendicitis is often difficult to diagnose in the young and the old, which often results in its late diagnosis in these age groups, with a concomitant increase in complications such as generalized peritonitis or abscess formation within the pelvis.

The colon can be the site of inflammatory bowel disease, either Crohn's or more commonly ulcerative colitis. The symptoms are abdominal pain with frequent diarrhoea and the passage of blood and mucus. An isolated part of the large bowel can be affected, but more often its entire length is involved, *panproctocolitis*. Medical treatment with anti-inflammatory drugs can control the disease. If these fail, it becomes fulminating when the entire large bowel has to be removed and the patient is left with an ileostomy, the terminal ileum being brought out as a spout through the abdominal wall over the right iliac fossa. Usually immediately after this operation the output from the terminal ileum is high, with considerable fluid loss. However, as time goes by the bowel seems to adjust to the absence of the colon, and the ileostomy becomes smaller in volume and less liquid. When ulcerative colitis lasts for several years, even with symptoms adequately controlled medically, panproctocolectomy is advisable, since ulcerative colitis predisposes to malignant change of the large bowel.

Coeliac disease (gluten enteropathy)

This is an immunological reaction to the gluten fraction of wheat which results in damage to the small intestinal mucosa with impaired absorptive capacity. Patients may present with features of malabsorption, excess stool fat with diarrhoea and weight loss, or they may be asymptomatic. The most common finding is anaemia due to folate or iron malabsorption, and when malabsorption is present it must be remembered that impaired absorption of vitamin K will impair blood clotting. Treatment involves the strict adherence to a gluten-free diet, and replacement of iron, folic acid and fat-soluble vitamins, e.g. vitamins D and K, may be necessary until the mucosa recovers.

Crohn's disease

This is a segmental inflammatory disease of unknown aetiology which involves all layers of the intestinal wall. The terminal ileum and caecum are most commonly involved but segmental inflammation may be found throughout the bowel and sometimes involves the oral cavity. Patients present with diarrhoea and/or abdominal pain. Sometimes patients develop intestinal obstruction, malabsorption (especially of vitamin B_{12}), and growth retardation when the disease develops before puberty. Extra-intestinal manifestations include arthritis and hepatobiliary disease.

Medical treatment includes the correction of malnutrition and suppression of the inflammatory process with corticosteroids. Other drugs including sulphasalazine, metronidazole and cytotoxics are occasionally helpful. In some patients localized disease is amenable to surgical excision. Management by bowel rest therapy involving prolonged intravenous nutrition or the use of elemental diets is currently undergoing evaluation.

Ulcerative colitis

This inflammatory disease of the intestine differs from Crohn's disease in three respects: the inflammation is confined to the mucosa, to the colon, and occurs in a continuous manner from the rectum to involve part or the whole of the large bowel. Depending on the extent of the disease, patients present with rectal bleeding or bloody diarrhoea. Severe disease presents abruptly with bloody diarrhoea and pyrexia. Complications include colonic perforation or haemorrhage, an increased incidence of colonic cancer after ten years, and extra-intestinal manifestations analogous to those seen in Crohn's disease.

Severe colitis requires vigorous treatment with high dose steroids, antibiotics, intravenous fluids and blood transfusions. Remission is induced by corticosteroids and maintained by sulphasalazine. Distal disease can be treated with steroid-containing enemas. The failure to respond to medical therapy or the development of pre-malignant changes requires surgical resection of both colon and rectum with the formation of an ileostomy.

Cancer of the intestine

Cancer usually arises in the rectum or colon. Although more usually a disease of middle and older age, it can occur in younger adults. Rectal cancer presents with the passage of fresh blood and sometimes mucus with the stool. Cancer involving the left colon can be responsible for a change in bowel habit (constipation alternating with diarrhoea), and right colonic cancer often presents late with iron deficiency anaemia. It can also present as anaemia from loss of blood into the lumen of the bowel, or as intestinal obstruction from mechanical blockage of the bowel by the growth. Unfortunately, by the time the diagnosis is made metastasis has often already occurred, particularly to the liver.

Diverticular disease

Small sacs of mucosa protrude through defects in a thickened muscle wall to form diverticula. The sigmoid colon is principally affected and the incidence of diverticula increases with age. Occlusion of the diverticula provokes inflammation, 'diverticulitis', which presents with pain in the left iliac fossa and pyrexia. Acute complications include perforation and abscess formation, and in the long-term diverticulitis may lead to progressive luminal narrowing with intestinal obstruction.

Acute episodes of diverticulitis are best treated with antibiotics and analgesics. Thereafter patients are advised to increase the bulk of their diet by the addition of bran. Occasionally, surgical resection may be needed.

Irritable bowel syndrome
This is one of the most common yet imprecise diagnostic labels applied in gastroenterological practice. It describes patients with some or all of the following symptoms: change of bowel habit, urgency and a feeling of incomplete evacuation, nausea and abdominal distension, abdominal pain; in whom conventional investigations have failed to identify a specific cause. Some patients appear to have a food intolerance, others respond to bulking agents such as bran and antispasmodics.

Infections of the gastrointestinal tract
Ingestion of viruses, bacteria or protozoa in contaminated water or food may lead to gastrointestinal infection and symptoms of diarrhoea and vomiting. Viral infections are usually mild and transient. Common bacterial infections include Salmonella and Campylobacter species, which are usually acquired from meat and poultry and are often associated with a profuse secretory diarrhoea. Protozoal infections include giardiasis, which may present with abdominal pain and ste-atorrhoea, and amoebiasis which can mimic ulcerative colitis. These infections are important partly because of the risk of transmission and mainly because of the consequent dehydration and eventual risk of pre-renal failure and electrolyte imbalance.

Treatment is by fluid and electrolyte replacement, usually orally, occasionally intravenously, particularly with protracted vomiting or severe dehydration. Anti-diarrhoeal drugs such as codeine phosphate and diphenoxylate hydrochloride (Lomotil) are potentially harmful. There is no indication for the routine use of antibiotics.

Intestinal obstruction
Intestinal obstruction may be caused by tumours, diverticular disease, Crohn's disease, adhesions or herniae. Symptoms include constipation, abdominal pain and distension, vomiting, and those of the primary disease. Surgical intervention is usually required, but

first the correction of any electrolyte imbalance or anaemia should be undertaken.

Anus

The anus, the lowest point of the alimentary tract, may give rise to several symptoms. Pain during defaecation can be due to acute fissure, which is a crack of the lining epithelium. This pain leads to spasm of the surrounding sphincter and tends to perpetuate the lesion. Treatment consists of dilating the tight muscle, under a general anaesthetic, so relaxing it and allowing the fissure to heal. Piles or haemorrhoids, which are excessive protruberances of the venous cushions or pads which normally make the anus continent of flatus, can cause itching, pain, bleeding and a sensation of something protruding from the anus. Treatment ranges from shrivelling the piles away by injecting sclerosant, to surgical ligature and removal. Just like the mouth, the anus can be the site of manifestations of systemic disorders such as venereal disease, Crohn's disease and can be infected with viruses producing wart-like *condylomata*.

Investigation of the intestine

The colon is investigated by means of sigmoidoscopy and barium enema: occasionally it is advantageous to inspect the entire mucosal lining by means of colonoscopy. Mucosal biopsies are easily obtained through the sigmoidoscope or colonoscope.

The small intestine is examined radiologically by duodenal intubation and the instillation of contrast media. Biopsies from the proximal jejunum can be obtained with the Crosby capsule, and the function of the distal ileum is assessed by the capacity for vitamin B_{12} absorption.

Occasionally it is necessary to establish a diagnosis of malabsorption by measuring the amount of fat excreted in the stool.

External hernia

This describes the protrusion of part of the bowel enclosed in a sac of peritoneum through the abdominal wall. Herniae may develop above or below the inguinal ligament (inguinal and femoral herniae respectively), through the umbilicus (umbilical hernia) or surgical scars in the abdominal wall (incisional hernia). The formation of herniae is encouraged by raised intra-abdominal pressure with heavy lifting or straining at stool, coughing or difficulty of micturition, and is particularly associated with liver cirrhosis and ascites. Sometimes the contents of the hernial sac become trapped and can no longer be pushed back into the abdomen, when obstruction and gangrene of the involved bowel may ensue.

Simple herniae can be managed by wearing a truss to prevent extrusion; larger or strangulated herniae require reduction and repair of the hernial orifice.

The liver
Viral hepatitis
Two of the viruses responsible for this disorder have been identified and labelled type A and type B. Other viruses await identification and are described as non-A non-B.

Type A hepatitis is transmitted by the faecal–oral route, hence its tendency to occur in epidemics and its old label of 'infectious hepatitis'. There is a transient viraemic phase at the onset of symptoms, which occurs 2–6 weeks after infection, and the virus is shed in the stool for one week before until one week after the onset of jaundice. Type A hepatitis can be diagnosed serologically. Type B hepatitis is transmitted by the parenteral and sexual routes, hence it used to be known as serum hepatitis. Drug addicts and male homosexuals are at particular risk. Clinical symptoms occur after an incubation period of 2–6 months, a viraemia may occur a few weeks before the onset of symptoms, and in contrast to type A hepatitis 10% of patients become chronic carriers. The hepatitis B virus (HBV) can now be identified by screening for the surface antigen (HBsAg). Patients who carry the 'e' antigen as well are especially infectious. An incomplete virus called the delta agent which depends on the presence of HBV may be transmitted in the same way and also produce a hepatitis syndrome. Non-A non-B viruses are transmitted parenterally, e.g. by blood transfusion. They are associated with a high incidence of chronic viraemia and chronic liver disease, and cannot yet be identified by serological markers.

The development of hepatitis is heralded by anorexia, lassitude, nausea and hepatic tenderness. After one or two weeks the patient becomes jaundiced and thereafter the symptoms and jaundice gradually subside. Two important complications may occur, acute liver failure, and the development of chronic hepatitis and cirrhosis. The former is associated with all types of hepatitis: chronic liver disease does not follow type A infections.

Hepatitis is important in dentistry because of the risk of acquiring or transmitting infection, especially the HBV. All blood and instruments contaminated with blood or saliva are dangerous. When treating high-risk patients the dentist is advised to wear gloves, a gown, mask and goggles. Used instruments should be placed on to tinfoil and care should be taken to avoid spraying saliva into the air; air turbine drills should not be used. After treatment, instruments are autoclaved, working surfaces washed down with sodium hypochlorite, and protective clothing disposed of. If a dentist pricks his skin with a contaminated instrument, hyperimmune globulin will confer protection. Active immunization to HBV is now available.

Chronic hepatitis
Chronic hepatitis may arise as a result of viral hepatitis, autoimmune disease, or alcohol abuse. Progress to cirrhosis frequently occurs. Patients may be jaundiced and develop liver failure. Those with autoimmune disease respond to corticosteroid therapy.

Cirrhosis
Cirrhosis is characterized by scarring and nodular regeneration which results in progressive deterioration in liver function with eventual liver failure, and increasing portal blood pressure with the development of spontaneous venous shunts such as oesophageal varices from which massive intestinal bleeding can occur. Alcohol abuse is the commonest cause of cirrhosis but this can also follow viral hepatitis or arise for no apparent reason. Management is usually confined to treating the effects of liver failure, except for rare disease such as haemochromatosis, in which removal of excess iron by venesection arrests the underlying liver damage.

Liver failure
Viral hepatitis and paracetamol overdose are the common causes of acute liver failure. Chronic liver failure may follow the development of cirrhosis for whatever reason.

Patients with liver failure develop jaundice. Impaired blood clotting reflects reduction in protein synthesis and impaired absorption of vitamin K, as a result of reduced bile flow and bile acid excretion. The accumulation of toxins impairs mental function, eventually patients become drowsy or comatose (*encephalopathy*) and hypoglycaemia may contribute to this problem. The accumulation of fluid in the peritoneal cavity (*ascites*) and gastrointestinal bleeding are both related to portal hypertension. Patients with acute liver failure suffer from vascular leakiness, hence pulmonary and cerebral oedema. The probability of impaired drug metabolism must be remembered in all patients with liver failure.

Principles of management include the use of aperients and lactulose to reduce toxin absorption and the tendency to encephalopathy. The maintenance of blood glucose, correction of clotting abnormalities, and avoidance of fluid overload, all require attention.

Patients with advanced liver disease and impending liver failure can be recognized by characteristic clinical features. Jaundice is best recognized in the conjunctiva. Ascites causes abdominal distension. They may have red palms, white nails, small telangiectatic blood vessels evident on the skin, and ankle oedema.

Liver tumours
The liver is a common site for metastases particularly from tumours of intestines and bronchus. Primary liver tumours are uncommon and usually develop in the context of chronic HBV infection or alcoholic cirrhosis.

Drugs and the liver
Many drugs are capable of causing liver damage. Chlorpromazine can lead to cholestasis, overdosage of paracetamol or halothane to hepatic necrosis, and methyldopa or isoniazid to chronic active hepatitis. Other drugs such as sulphonamides may render the patient jaundiced either because of hepatitis or haemolysis. It is also important to remember that liver damage is associated with impaired drug metabolism; this applies particularly to lipid-soluble drugs which require conjugation.

Jaundice
Jaundice may occur because of *haemolysis*, liver disease (*hepatocellular*) e.g. hepatitis or cirrhosis, or *obstruction* of the bile duct. Bile duct obstruction is most commonly associated with gallstones or pancreatic disease. In haemolytic jaundice, excess urobilinogen is present in the urine, whereas in obstructive jaundice there is no urobilinogen or urobilin in the urine.

Occasionally gallstones leave the gallbladder and lodge in the common bile duct when severe central abdominal pain is followed by the development of jaundice.

The common bile duct may be compressed by the enlargement of the pancreas on account of malignancy or pancreatitis. In addition to jaundice, such patients suffer from weight loss and abdominal pain which radiates to the back. Endocrine and exocrine pancreatic insufficiency respectively cause diabetes and malabsorption with steatorrhoea.

Bile duct obstruction due to pancreatic carcinoma or gallstones usually requires surgery; pancreatitis may resolve with conservative management.

Investigations of the liver and biliary system

The ideal liver function test does not exist, and patients with suspected hepatobiliary disease must be investigated using a combination of techniques. Ultrasonography is useful in demonstrating intrahepatic tumours and identifying obstructive jaundice. It will usually show dilated bile ducts into which contrast medium can be injected directly with a fine needle (*percutaneous transhepatic cholangiography*) and frequently disclose a cause. Severe hepatic damage correlates best with abnormalities of prothrombin time which does not correct with vitamin K (in contrast to that associated with cholestasis and malabsorption). Active hepatic necrosis such as occurs in viral hepatitis results in striking elevation of the serum enzymes, and when viral-related liver disease is suspected, HBsAg should be sought.

When planning anaesthesia and surgery on jaundiced patients, important precautions are necessary as outlined in Chapter 1. These include the correction of any coagulation defect by preoperative parenteral vitamin K injections, the preoperative boosting of urine output to prevent renal failure, and in obstructive jaundice the use of prophylactic antibacterial therapy, since bile in an obstructed duct is likely to contain micro-organisms. Vitamin C should also be given since jaundice depletes the liver stores of this nutrient which is essential for wound healing.

Symptoms of gastrointestinal disease

Dysphagia

Progressive dysphagia for solids is typical of oesophageal carcinoma, intermittent dysphagia with preceding heartburn may denote peptic oesophagitis with stricture. Patients with achalasia often have more difficulty swallowing liquids than solids.

Vomiting
This is a feature of raised intracranial pressure, gastroenteritis, pyloric obstruction due to peptic ulcer or carcinoma, or small bowel obstruction.

Haematemesis
The vomiting of blood follows bleeding from oesophageal varices or mucosal tears (which are caused by prolonged retching: Mallory–Weiss syndrome), gastric or duodenal ulcers or erosions. Frequent bleeding from the stomach or duodenum occurs in the absence of vomiting, the blood is altered as it passes through the intestine to emerge from the rectum as black tarry material (melaena).

Diarrhoea
Acute diarrhoea may be caused by drugs such as antibiotics, or by infections such as salmonella gastroenteritis. More chronic diarrhoea may signify inflammatory bowel disease such as Crohn's disease or ulcerative colitis, disease causing partial obstruction such as hernia, diverticular disease or tumours, or any cause of malabsorption.

Malabsorption
This is usually characterized by fat malabsorption which presents with offensive bulky stool. It is particularly associated with pancreatic exocrine insufficiency, but also occurs with coeliac disease, Crohn's disease, and small intestinal bacterial growth.

Abdominal pain
Upper abdominal pain occurs in patients with peptic ulcer disease, pancreatic and gallbladder disease. The pain of peptic ulcer disease is epigastric and relieved by eating, in pancreatic disease it radiates to the back. Central abdominal pain occurs with small bowel disease, e.g. obstruction, and lower abdominal pain with colonic disease.

Generalized abdominal pain associated with rigidity of the abdominal wall and absent bowel sounds denotes peritonitis. This is usually caused by a perforated viscus due to an ulcer or diverticulitis and constitutes a surgical emergency.

The significance of gastrointestinal disease to dentists
Some patients with gastrointestinal disease may present to the dentist with oral lesions, e.g. Crohn's disease, and many others will have

other clues to the presence of underlying intestinal disease, e.g. aphthous ulcers in patients with coeliac disease. Patients with all forms of intestinal disease are liable to lose blood and ultimately become anaemic, posing an anaesthetic risk. Those with malabsorption not only develop anaemia because of impaired absorption of haematinics, but are also liable to bleed excessively because of the reduced absorption of vitamin K. A significant number of patients with liver disease and jaundice carry the HBV virus. Some have significant impairment of blood coagulation and drug metabolism. Finally, corticosteroids are used to treat inflammatory bowel disease and some forms of chronic liver disease: such patients may need additional steroid cover for procedures requiring anaesthesia. *See also* hepatic disease, p.297.

11 Diabetes mellitus and other endocrine disorders

DIABETES MELLITUS

Diabetes mellitus can most usefully be regarded as a term to describe a series of separate conditions characterized by a chronically raised blood glucose level. Elevation of the blood glucose is known as *hyperglycaemia* and is associated with a number of characteristic symptoms:

Thirst (polydipsia),

Passing large quantities of urine (polyuria) due to the osmotic effect of the glucose which it contains,

Tiredness and listlessness,

Loss of weight due to breakdown of body protein and fat.

Glucose in the urine may lead to vulvo-vaginal itching in females and balanitis in males and may predispose to superadded monilial infection.

The symptoms of severe thirst and polyuria are unmistakable in overt diabetes and are associated with an elevated blood glucose level. However, there is a 'grey area' where blood glucose values fall short of frank diabetes but are abnormal when the patient is administered glucose by mouth. This is the glucose tolerance test (GTT) and it helps to distinguish these two groups. Patients with intermittent glycosuria or who have casual or fasting blood glucose values in the equivocal range are described as having 'impaired glucose tolerance'.

About 1–2% of the population of western countries are known diabetics. The incidence however is gradually rising for all types of diabetes.

Classification

Diabetes mellitus is now conveniently divided into two main types:

1. *Insulin-dependent diabetes (IDD)* or *Type I* diabetes (previously known as juvenile onset diabetes).
2. *Non insulin-dependent diabetes (NIDD)* or *Type II* diabetes (previously known as maturity onset diabetes).

Both may be regarded as primary diabetes mellitus. Secondary diabetes mellitus is much less common and is associated with:

Loss of insulin-producing β-cells by surgery or destructive diseases of the pancreas, and

Other hormonal disorders such as Cushing's syndrome (including steroid therapy), acromegaly and thyrotoxicosis. Some women may become transiently diabetic during the later months of pregnancy (gestational diabetes).

Table 3   Clinical features of IDD and NIDD.

	Insulin-dependent diabetes	Non insulin-dependent diabetes
Age	Children and young adults	Mainly middle age and over
Sex	Male = female	Male < female
Proportion of all diabetics	35%	65%
Onset	Acute or subacute	Gradual (months or even years)
Symptoms	Present and may be severe at diagnosis	Often absent or slight. Sometimes diagnosis is a chance finding.
Weight loss	Marked	Slow or absent
Ketosis	Common	Absent
Plasma insulin level	Absent or low	May be lowered or normal —often raised particularly in the obese
Insulin receptor sensitivity	Sensitive	Often relatively insulin resistant

Aetiology

Many pathogenic mechanisms may be involved in producing the two types of diabetes. In *insulin-dependent diabetes* the following factors are important:

A genetically susceptible person (certain histocompatability antigens are positively associated with IDD),

An immune reaction to pancreatic islet cells (islet cell antibody),

A 'trigger' mechanism to stimulate the immune reaction (virus infection seems most likely).

In *non insulin-dependent diabetes:*
Genetic susceptibility plays a more important role than in IDD,
Obesity is a major factor.

Complications of diabetes
It is now clear that good diabetic control is at least one but not the only important factor in avoiding long-term complications. They do not ususally appear before 10 years of diabetes. Only 40% of insulin-dependent diabetics survive 40 years or more from the time of diagnosis.

The major complications may reflect a specific effect on small blood vessels (*microangiopathy*).

Eye disease
Retinopathy (haemorrhages, exudates and new vessel formation),
Diabetic retinopathy is the commonest cause of blindness between the ages 30–64 years,
Regular ophthalmoscopy and laser photocoagulation have considerably improved the outlook.

Renal damage
A specific glomerular sclerosis occurs in diabetes,
In the initial stage it normally manifests as protein in the urine,
This may progress to renal failure (approximately 75% of patients are in terminal renal failure after 10 years of continuous proteinuria).

Nerve damage (neuropathy)
Diabetic neuropathy usually affects the extremities and is normally sensory,
Patients complain of pain, pins and needles (*paraesthesiae*) or of loss of sensation.
However, a motor neuropathy also occurs; typically giving rise to muscle weakness.

Occasionally longstanding diabetes is associated with *autonomic neuropathy* which gives rise to postural hypotension, gastric distension, nocturnal diarrhoea, gustatory sweating, urinary retention and a number of other manifestations of autonomic nervous system dysfunction.

Diabetic gangrene
Typically digital gangrene occurs in the feet as a result of a combination of ischaemia, sensory loss and infection.

The effects of diabetes leads to premature atheroma of large arteries. Diabetics are particularly prone to:
   Premature death from myocardial infarction,
   Features of peripheral vascular disease.

Treatment

Control of diet is necessary in all diabetics. In some non insulin-dependent diabetics it is all that is required to restore glucose tolerance. It is essential that the major part of carbohydrate consumed should not be in the form of refined sugar. Carbohydrate foods rich in dietary fibre are absorbed more slowly and so are preferable. Generally there has been a trend towards a diet high in fibre and low in fat for all types of diabetes.

In insulin-dependent diabetes the energy content is decided on the basis of the physical activity of the patient. The carbohydrate content which is normally about 50% is divided into 10 g portions and is spread throughout the main meals and snacks of the day to coincide with the peak of action of the administered insulins.

In non insulin-dependent diabetes dietary restriction is usually designed to achieve weight loss in the obese.

Insulin is essential in ketosis prone insulin-dependent diabetics. It may also be required by some non insulin-dependent diabetics who remain inadequately controlled on oral hypoglycaemic drugs. The majority of insulins are derived from pigs and are low in antigenicity. Recently synthetic human insulins have become available but do not appear to have clear advantages over highly purified pig insulins.

Clinically insulins can be classified as follows:
   Short-acting,
   Medium-acting,
   Long-acting.
In the elderly where less than perfect control is acceptable and in patients changing from oral hypoglycaemic drugs to insulin, a single injection of a long-acting insulin may be satisfactory, e.g. Ultratard or Lentard insulin (insulin zinc suspensions).

However, in the young insulin-dependent diabetic the aim of therapy is to achieve the best possible control. At least two injections per day of insulin are necessary, usually of a mixture of a short-and medium-acting insulin, e.g.
   Actrapid and Monotard, i.e. a neutral insulin plus an insulin zinc suspension.

Velosulin and Insulatard, i.e. a neutral insulin plus an isophane insulin. (Fig. 9)

Control is assessed by using Diastix or an alternative urine test strip to check the urine for glucose before each main meal and before bedtime. More precisely the blood glucose can be measured at home on a finger-prick specimen using reagent sticks and a glucose colorimeter.

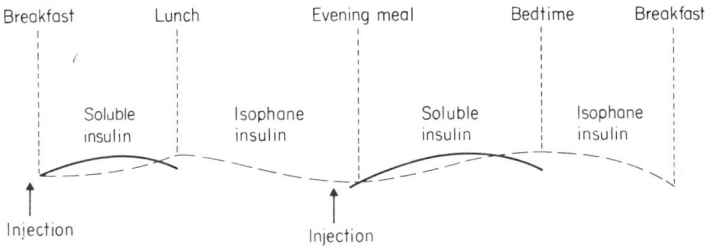

Fig. 9 Typical insulin regime.

With a scale of insulin doses, patients are able to alter the dose of the appropriate insulin up or down as circumstances demand:
1. Infection may lead to hyperglycaemia and ketoacidosis if insulin doses are not increased,
2. Reduced food intake may lead to hypoglycaemia,
3. Exercise may lower the blood glucose.

Oral hypoglycaemic agents. Dietary restriction of carbohydrate or change to unrefined carbohydrate foods is the cornerstone of therapy in the non insulin-dependent diabetic. However, as many as 50% of such patients are not adequately controlled on diet or are unable to comply with dietary restriction. When such measures fail oral hypoglycaemic drugs may be useful.

Sulphonylureas such as glibenclamide and glipizide have replaced the first generation drug chlorpropamide. They act by stimulating insulin release and increasing insulin receptor sensitivity. Consequently they are prone to produce *hypoglycaemia*. They are particularly appropriate in patients who are not obese (their use is normally associated with weight gain).

Biguanides such as metformin act by inhibiting gastrointestinal carbohydrate absorption and by enhancing peripheral glucose utilization. They do not have their action through insulin release and therefore *do not* cause hypoglycaemia. They are particularly appropriate for obese patients and tend to potentiate weight loss.

Diabetic ketoacidosis
This is due to acute insulin deficiency which may result from:
1. Error in dosage (mistaken or occasionally deliberate),
2. Increase in insulin requirement (at times of acute stress, e.g.
   infection, surgery, etc.),
3. Initial presentation of insulin-dependent diabetes.
In dental practice there are two particular risk situations:
(a) Missing the morning insulin injection (or lowering the dose) to
    accommodate fasting for general anaesthesia (p.298).
(b) Post-surgery reduction of insulin dosage because of the inability
    to eat (carbohydrate should be taken in the form of sugary drinks).
Insulin-dependent diabetics are clearly more prone to ketoacidosis
because typically they lack endogenous insulin. A severe state of
tissue breakdown occurs in which high levels of catecholamines,
glucocorticoids and glucagon play a part. Hyperglycaemia leads to
dehydration, ketonuria to loss of cations, and cellular breakdown
to negative nitrogen balance (p. 12).
    Clinically the onset is slow over hours or days with the develop-
ment of:
        Thirst,
        Polyuria,
        Dehydration,
        Vomiting and abdominal pain.
Drowsiness and deep sighing respiration may be the result of severe
acidaemia.

Treatment, which should be undertaken in hospital, consists of:
    Replacement of fluid and electrolytes:
        Saline with potassium supplementation is given intravenously,
        The patient may require up to 5–6 l of fluid in the first few
        hours of treatment.
    Replacement of insulin:
        Continuously through an infusion pump,
        Or by regular small doses given subcutaneously.
The use of bicarbonate to correct acidosis is not now felt to be important and there may be inherent dangers in too rapid correction
of the acid–base status.
    Currently doctors encourage self-adjustment of insulin regimes to
cope with control difficulties. This has resulted in a reduced incidence
of ketoacidosis.

Hypoglycaemia

Symptoms of hypoglycaemia occur at a blood glucose level of less than about 2 mmol/l. However, symptoms can occasionally occur at higher levels, particularly in the elderly, but also in circumstances in which the blood glucose level has fallen rapidly.

In insulin-dependent diabetes hypoglycaemia may result from:

> Too little to eat,
> Delay in taking a meal,
> Unusual or heavy exertion,
> Error in insulin dosage.

Hypoglycaemia may occur about 3–6 hours after the administration of modern sulphonylurea agents and can occasionally be prolonged and life-threatening.

The symptoms of hypoglycaemia can be divided into:

1. Those due to inadequate glucose for brain function (*neuroglycopenia*),
2. Those associated with the secondary release of catecholamines.

Neuroglycopenic symptoms:

> double vision or blurring of vision,
> facial paraesthesiae,
> ataxia (staggering),
> mood changes,
> difficulty in concentration,
> fits,
> loss of consciousness.

Prolonged severe neuroglycopenia may lead to permanent brain damage.

Sympathometic symptoms:

> sweating,
> palpitations,
> tremor,
> pallor,
> dilatation of pupils,
> headache.

Management

In conscious patients Dextrosol glucose tablets, sweet tea or glucose drinks can be administered. Even when the patient is drowsy, honey can be rubbed around the gums and cheeks.

In the unconscious or uncooperative patient 25–50% glucose solution can be injected intravenously or glucagon can be administered intramuscularly (the latter may be particularly of value in an aggressive patient).

On recovery the patient must be given a further 20 g of carbohydrate by mouth.

Surgery and anaesthesia in diabetic patients

There are two important considerations:

Is the patient insulin-dependent?

How long will the patient be prevented from taking food by mouth?

In patients who are controlled by diet alone no special precautions are usually necessary except that the urine should be checked regularly for glucose after operation.

In patients taking oral hypoglycaemic drugs

Omit the drug on the day of operation for minor surgery,

Treat as for insulin-dependent diabetes if major surgery is contemplated.

In insulin-dependent diabetics

When major surgery and general anaesthesia is contemplated:

Admit to hospital 24–48 hours prior to surgery,

Achieve control by multiple injections of short-acting insulin,

On the day of operation infuse 500 ml of 5–10% dextrose with 10 units of insulin over 4 hours,

The rate of insulin infusion can be adjusted according to the blood glucose values checked on a reflectancemeter.

This regime can be continued until feeding is reinstated after surgery, which if elective should be done as early in the day as possible.

Note. Beware of the trend in past years to reduce or miss the insulin dose on the morning of operation, but remember that the greatest danger is from intraoperative hypoglycaemia.

Susceptibility to infections

Poor control of diabetes mellitus is assocated with a lowered resistance to infection. The development of a *carbuncle* (a necrotizing infection of the skin and subcutaneous tissue with multiple formed or incipient sinuses) may unmask latent diabetes or even precipitate ketoacidotic coma. Diabetics who have unexplained weight loss, symptoms of pulmonary disease or an increase in their insulin requirements may have contracted *pulmonary tuberculosis*. All newly diagnosed diabetics should have a chest radiograph performed. Resistant glycosuria favours the development of *urinary tract infections* and similarly it is often associated with *pruritus vulvae* caused by *candidosis*. *Oral candidosis* may also be an early, though not specific, sign of uncontrolled diabetes as may severe, chronic *periodontal disease*, though this is seldom gross in those with well-controlled diabetes.

DISORDERS OF THE THYROID

Hyperthyroidism—thyrotoxicosis
Hypothyroidism—myxoedema
Thyroid swelling—goitre

Hyperthyroidism
This condition results from overactivity of the thyroid gland and an excess of the circulating thyroid hormones thyroxine (T4) and triiodothyronine (T3). Usually the levels of both hormones are raised, however occasionally only triiodothyronine is secreted in excess. This condition is called *T3 toxicosis*.

Effects of excess thyroid hormones
Thyroid hormones increase the metabolism of the body. The most important *symptoms* are nervousness and anxiety, sweating and intolerance of heat and weight loss despite an increased appetite. The patient may also complain of breathlessness, palpitations, tiredness and frequent bowel motions. On examination the most important *signs* are rapid pulse rate, hot moist skin, tremor of outstretched hands, a diffuse thyroid swelling (Grave's disease) and retraction of the eyelids giving a 'pop-eye' appearance.

In the most common form of hyperthyroidism (*Grave's disease*) the eye signs are frequently more severe than simple lid retraction, with swelling of the contents of the orbit pushing the eye forward (*exophthalmos*). Involvement of the extraocular muscles may give rise to double vision and abnormalities of eye movement (*ophthalmoplegia*).

Hyperthyroid Grave's disease is one of the commonest endocrine disorders. It is six times more common in women that in men and it normally occurs between the ages of 30 and 50.

Diffuse thyroid enlargement and overactivity is the result of stimulation by an IgG autoantibody (thyroid stimulating immunoglobulin—TSI). The associated eye signs are believed to be the result of a separate stimulating immunoglobulin and will not necessarily respond to treatment of the primary thyroid condition. *Ophthalmic Grave's disease* relates to isolated exophthalmos and/or ophthalmoplegia occurring in the absence of thyrotoxicosis.

'Masked' or 'apathetic' hyperthyroidism is particularly common in the elderly. Cardiovascular features such as atrial fibrillation (which may revert to sinus rhythm after treatment) or cardiac failure may predominate. In such cases the thyroid gland may be irregularly enlarged due to a *multinodular goitre.*

Thyroid crisis. Doctors are now more aware of the features of thyrotoxicosis and this has resulted in earlier diagnosis and treatment. Rarely however rapid acceleration of hyperthyroidism still occurs. The patient develops a marked increase in the pulse rate, cardiac failure, hyperthermia and physical and mental exhaustion.

Diagnosis
Determination of the serum thyroxine level is the simplest test. The serum triiodothyronine level is also elevated and in T3 toxicosis may be elevated by itself. More sophisticated tests are now available when direct measurement of serum hormone levels are not confirmatory. The TRH test, for example, measures the ability of the anterior pituitary to release thyroid stimulating hormone (TSH). This will be impaired when the anterior pituitary is suppressed by 'negative feedback' of high circulating thyroid hormone levels.

Management
The aim of treatment is to decrease the amount of hormone produced by the thyroid.
1. *Antithyroid drugs* decrease the synthesis of thyroid hormone,
2. *Radioactive iodine* is taken up by thyroid cells and causes damage resulting in a permanent decrease in activity,
3. *Surgery* reduces the amount of functioning thyroid tissue.

β–*adrenergic blocking drugs* such as propranolol may be used to achieve rapid control of clinical features of hyperthyroidism. They do not reduce output of hormone but they block the peripheral adrenergic effects. They are particularly useful in preventing thyroid crisis, as preparation for thyroid surgery, to achieve control whilst awaiting the therapeutic effect of radioiodine and as an adjunct to antithyroid drugs.

Antithyroid drugs. Carbimazole and propylthiouracil block thyroid hormone production at different points in its synthesis. These drugs require to be given for at least one year until natural remission of the primary thyroid condition occurs. They are used particularly during the childbearing years and during pregnancy. About 50% of patients relapse within one year of stopping therapy. A small proportion of patients develop skin rashes. Rarely agranulocytosis may occur which presents with sore throat, usually within the first few weeks of therapy.

Radioactive iodine. ^{131}I treatment is particularly indicated in patients past childbearing years, following unsuccessful control of thyrotoxicosis after partial thyroidectomy, and to achieve ablation of thyroid activity in patients with cardiac complications or other serious medical conditions.

The response tends to be slow, and control using antithyroid drugs is usually necessary as a temporary measure until it is attained.

The vast majority of patients eventually become hypothyroid after radioiodine and require thyroxine replacement.

Surgery is an effective and rapid means of achieving control. It is particularly indicated in young patients who relapse off antithyroid drugs, when thyrotoxicosis is associated with a large goitre, in patients with a single toxic nodule and in patients who are unwilling to take drugs.

In skilled hands partial thyroidectomy is a safe procedure particularly with the use of antithyroid drugs and β-adrenoceptor blocking drugs preoperatively. Rarely damage to the recurrent laryngeal nerve at operation gives rise to hoarseness, or mistaken removal of the parathyroid glands results in hypocalcaemia and symptoms of tetany after operation.

Hypothyroidism
This condition results from decreased function of the thyroid gland and a decreased level of circulating thyroid hormones. A mucoid

substance is deposited in the skin and other tissues in the body which is called 'myxoedema'. Women are affected five times more frequently than men. It occurs at all ages but peaks at 40–60 years of age.

Causes of hypothyroidism

Primary failure of the thyroid gland may be due to destructive treatment for hyperthyroidism, autoimmune destruction (*Hashimoto's thyroiditis*), inherited enzyme defects of the thyroid gland (*dyshormonogenesis*), iodine deficiency or goitrogenic substances.

Secondary hypothroidism is due to failure of TSH production by the pituitary gland. This is much less common than primary hypothyroidism.

Clinical features
Two factors are involved: lack of thyroid hormone causing cellular metabolism to slow down and the effects of localized accumulation of mucoprotein. The onset of hypothyroidism may be slow and the clinical features may go unnoticed. The most important symptoms are tiredness and lethargy, cold intolerance, mental slowness, dryness of skin and hair and weight gain. In addition, patients may complain of constipation, menstrual dysfunction, hoarseness, a sensation of pins and needles in the hands, deteriorating memory, deafness and muscle cramps. Occasionally patients may present with the symptoms of ischaemic heart disease, which may occur prematurely in long-standing hypothyroidism. There may be a history of other autoimmune conditions, such as pernicious anaemia or rheumatoid arthritis.

   Important clinical signs include a dry scaly skin which is cold and thickened, puffiness and pallor of the face (particularly periorbital), dry, lack-lustre hair, slowing of the pulse and a delayed relaxation phase of the Achilles tendon jerk.

Diagnosis
Diagnosis can be confirmed by a low serum thyroxine level. In primary hypothyroidism the anterior pituitary gland produces an excess of TSH to attempt to compensate for low thyroid hormone levels. A high basal TSH level consolidates the diagnosis since a

lowered T4 level can be confusingly low in the elderly or chronically sick and does not necessarily indicate hypothyroidism.

Treatment
Thyroxine can be taken orally once daily. In patients with recent onset of hypothroidism the dose can be raised to full replacement levels of 0.15–0.2 mg daily fairly quickly. However, in the elderly, in patients with long-standing hypothyroidism, or in the presence of established ischaemic heart disease the dose must be started at low levels and increased very slowly over a number of months to avoid precipitating symptoms of myocardial ischaemia or precipitating heart failure.

Myxoedema coma
This is an uncommon but important complication of hypothyroidism. It is particularly exacerbated by hypothermia, but drugs such as narcotics and anaesthetics contribute to its development in pre-existing hypothyroidism.

Thyroid swelling (goitre)
Goitres may present as:
    Diffuse enlargement,
    Multiple nodules,
    Solitary nodule.

Thyroid swellings can be differentiated from those lying outside the gland by the fact that they move upwards on swallowing.

The patient with diffuse goitre may be:
1. *Hyperthyroid (Grave's disease).* Occasionally subacute, viral thyroiditis gives rise to transient thyrotoxicosis and painful thyroid swelling;
2. *Hypothyroid (Hashimoto's thyroiditis).* In this case thyroid swelling results from chronic TSH stimulation of a failing thyroid. Dyshormonogenesis results in a large goitre;
3. *In a normal thyroid state;* or have a
4. *Colloid (or simple) goitre* (commonly seen in adolescence and pregnancy).

Note.In the early stages Hasimoto's thyroiditis may not give rise to hypothyroidism.

Multinodular goitres are common in the elderly. They occasionally lead to thyrotoxicosis. They are rarely malignant.

Single thyroid nodules may be:
(a) Functioning (hot nodule). These may give rise to T3 toxicosis. They are seldom malignant.
(b) Non-functioning (cold nodule). These may be solid and are sometimes malignant. They may be cystic and these are only occasionally malignant.

Investigation
Serum T4 and T3 values together with a basal TSH level provide information about the functional status of the gland. Thyroid auto-antibodies are present in the majority of patients with autoimmune thyroiditis. Radioisotope scanning and ultrasound scanning help to define the structural features of the goitre.

Treatment
In goitres produced by TSH stimulation, suppression of TSH by thyroxine therapy often gives rise to regression of thyroid swelling. In the majority of other goitres surgical intervention may be necessary to reduce the hormonal output of the gland, to relieve pressure symptoms from the gland or to rule out malignancy in the thyroid swelling.

Note. Patients with autoimmune thyroiditis rarely develop carcinoma of the thyroid, however, the affected gland is occasionally the seat of a lymphoma in later life.

PITUITARY GLAND

Anatomy and physiology
The pituitary gland is situated in the sella turcica which is bridged above by the diaphragma sella. Important anatomical relationships include the sphenoid air cells below and anteriorly, the optic chiasma

above and the cavernous sinus on either side. The anterior lobe of
the pituitary secretes growth hormone (GH), thyrotrophic hormone
(TSH), adrenocorticotrophic hormone (ACTH), follicle stimulating
hormone (FSH), luteinizing hormone (LH) and prolactin (Prl). The
posterior lobe secretes antidiuretic hormone (ADH) and oxytocin.
The anterior pituitary hormones are controlled by releasing and
inhibitory peptides released by the hypothalamus into small blood
vessels which link the hypothalamus with the pituitary via its stalk.
ADH and oxytocin are released from pituitary nerve endings whose
neurones reside in the hypothalamus.

Pituitary tumours
Pituitary tumours produce their effects in three ways:
1. Specific hypersecretion of one or more pituitary hormones.
   (Table 4).

Table 4   Pituitary hormone hypersecretion.

Hypersecretion	Name of condition
Prolactin	Prolactinoma
GH	Acromegaly (known as gigantism if prepubertal)
ACTH	Cushing's disease
TSH (rare)	TSHoma (produces hyperthyroidism)
No obvious secretion	Non-functioning tumour

2. Expansion of the tumour compresses the surrounding normal
   pituitary producing a deficiency of some or all of the other pituitary
   hormones.
3. The tumour can erode into the air sinuses and the cavernous
   sinus. This can result in headache and cranial nerve defects.
   Expansion of the tumour out of the fossa can encroach upon the
   optic chiasma resulting in visual field defects.

Prolactinoma
This is the commonest pituitary tumour and mainly occurs in women.
It has to be distinguished from physiological hypersecretion of
prolactin which occurs in pregnancy, lactation and stressful situations
and from drug-induced hyperprolactinaemia which occurs with the

antihypertensive drugs methyldopa and reserpine, oestrogens, phenothiazines and metoclopramide. The prolactin hypersecretion in females produces breast milk secretion (galactorrhoea), menstrual irregularities and infertility. In males, it usually presents as a rapidly expanding tumour associated with hypopituitarism, headaches, visual field defects and occasionally galactorrhoea.

Diagnosis. Confirmed by the measurement of serum prolactin. High-resolution CAT scan often clearly delineates the tumour and its encroachment upon surrounding structures.

Treatment. Bromocriptine, a dopamine agonist, is effective in reducing prolactin hypersecretion and in shrinking most of the tumours. As the tumours can rapidly re-expand once bromocriptine is stopped, surgical resection, external radiotherapy or radioisotope implantation are often advised for large tumours.

Acromegaly
This results from excessive secretion of GH. If this occurs prior to puberty before the skeletal epiphyses have fused, elongation of the skeleton occurs and the condition is called 'gigantism'. If it occurs after puberty, height is not affected but the tissues thicken, the condition being called 'acromegaly'. The patient often presents with excessive sweating, extreme lethargy, progressive coarsening of the features and enlargement of the hands, feet and head. Enlargement of the jaw results in an overriding bite, separation of the molar teeth and ill-fitting dentures. The buccal mucosa becomes thickened and the tongue large and coarse. Diabetes mellitus and hypertension are important complications. Without treatment, cardiac sequelae are eventually fatal.

Diagnosis. Confirmed by measuring GH in response to a glucose load. In normal subjects GH is suppressed by glucose, whereas in acromegaly there is a paradoxical rise in GH. Radiology may show the enlarged lower jaw, prominent frontal ridges, enlarged air sinuses and often enlargement of the pituitary fossa. High-resolution CAT scan will delineate the tumour. Visual field charting will show any encroachment on the optic chiasma.

Treatment. Surgical removal is the treatment most often advocated but external radiotherapy or radioisotope implantation is also effective.

Bromocriptine does reduce the serum GH in some. Since it is only moderately effective, it is not usually used as the sole form of treatment but mainly as an adjunct to external radiotherapy which by itself can take some years to normalize GH.

Cushing's disease

This refers to excess adrenal glucocorticoid (mainly cortisol) secretion as the result of a pituitary tumour releasing ACTH. Cushing's syndrome refers to cortisol hypersecretion as the result of an adrenal adenoma, carcinoma or from tumours producing ectopic ACTH (i.e. outwith the pituitary). Ectopic ACTH secretion most often comes from tumours of the lung but tumours involving the thymus, pancreas and gut (carcinoid tumours) may be implicated. The characteristic appearance of glucocorticoid hypersecretion is that of truncal obesity, a moon-shaped, reddened face and thin arms and legs due to muscle wasting. To distinguish early Cushing's from simple obesity one should look for the four cardinal signs of Cushing's, namely thinning of the skin, proximal myopathy, temporal balding of the scalp hair and oedema of the conjunctiva (known as chemosis). The oedema and hypertension are caused by fluid retention. Diabetes mellitus often occurs. Stretching of the thin skin produces striae which have a violet hue due to the underlying vasculature and are found over the abdomen, thorax and thighs. The thin skin also results in easy bruising. Features of virilism may occur if the adrenal also hypersecretes adrenal androgens producing hirsutism, frontal balding and acne. The excess circulating cortisol produces profound muscle wasting and also osteoporosis of the bones. The latter results in collapse of the vertebrae producing kyphosis and also fractures of other bones especially the ribs. Psychological changes, e.g. depression, psychosis, can be severe and can even result in suicide.

Diagnosis. Confirmed by measuring urinary free cortisol which is elevated in Cushing's. High-dose dexamethasone suppression, metyrapone stimulation of ACTH and basal ACTH measurements are used to discriminate the cause of Cushing's. CAT scan is used nowadays to locate the tumour.

Treatment. This depends on the aetiology:
1. Pituitary ACTH tumour: radioactive implantation or surgical resection.
2. Adrenal adenoma and carcinoma: surgical removal of the tumour. Aminoglutethimide, metyrapone and o,p^{1}DDD (Metotane), a

cytotoxic agent which selectively inhibits adrenal cortical activity, are used to inhibit an unresectable primary carcinoma and any secondaries.
3. Ectopic ACTH secretion: surgical resection of the ectopic ACTH secreting tumour: if this cannot be found then bilateral adrenalectomy.

Nelson's syndrome

In the past bilateral adrenalectomy was advocated for pituitary-dependent Cushing's. This meant that the tumour remained in the pituitary fossa and over years enlarged, causing local trouble. The prolonged hypersecretion of ACTH produced pigmentation resembling that in Addison's disease (*see* below), the condition being called 'Nelson's syndrome'.

Treatment. Surgical resection, radioisotope implantation, external radiotherapy and sodium valproate (an anti-epileptic drug).

Hypopituitarism

This often results from destruction of the pituitary gland as the result of an expanding tumour. Hypopituitarism can also result from pituitary ischaemia following post-partum haemorrhage, whereas trauma can sever the pituitary stalk producing functional hypopituitarism. Hypopituitarism results in secondary failure of the thyroid, adrenal and reproductive glands. The patient becomes lethargic, nauseated, loses sexual hair (axillary, pubic and beard growth) and becomes impotent. Diabetes insipidus (*see* below) may also occur.

Diagnosis. Confirmed by dynamic tests of pituitary function.

Treatment. Replacement with thyroxine, hydrocortisone, sex hormones and ADH (given as DDAVP—desmopressin, an ADH [vasopressin] analogue—as a nasal spray).

Diabetes insipidus

This results from lack of ADH following destruction of the posterior pituitary, pituitary stalk or median eminence of the hypothalamus. This results in an inability to concentrate urine. The patient has profound polyuria, nocturia and thirst.

Diagnosis. In a normal person, water deprivation for 8 h causes urine volume to decrease and the urine to become more concentrated, (i.e. its osmolality rises). This does not occur in those with diabetes insipidus.

Treatment. ADH is replaced by the analogue DDAVP which is given as a nasal spray.

Adrenocortical insufficiency
This can result from:
1. Lack of ACTH secretion.
2. Adrenal gland failure (known as Addison's disease).
3. Sudden cessation of steroid replacement or steroid therapy, where this has resulted in adrenal atrophy.

Addison's disease
This is most often caused by a disturbed immune reaction (autoimmunity) which destroys the adrenal glands. Other causes which are now rarely seen are tuberculosis, metastases and haemorrhage. The patient develops profound weight loss, anorexia, vomiting, diarrhoea and weakness. The low serum cortisol and corticosterone (i.e. the glucocorticoids) result in a reduced feedback onto the pituitary, hence ACTH secretion rises and hyperpigmentation occurs. The pigmentation can be distinguished from sunburn for it is found on the buccal mucosa, gums, palmar creases, pressure areas, e.g. belt area, bra straps, and over bony prominences such as knees, elbows and knuckles. Due to the lack of the mineralocorticoid hormone, aldosterone, serum electrolytes are disturbed with low sodium, high potassium and elevated urea.

Diagnosis. Confirmed by a lack of rise of serum cortisol to ACTH injection.

Treatment. This should be vigorously treated for the condition can be rapidly fatal. Salt loss should be corrected by intravenous saline. The glucocorticoids are replaced with hydrocortisone and aldosterone by fludrocortisone. The usual replacement regimen is:
(a) Hydrocortisone 20 mg in the morning and 10 mg in late afternoon.
(b) Fludrocortisone 0.1–0.2 mg each morning.

Stressful events. The patient should carry a card stating the diagnosis and the name, address and telephone number of the physician from whom medical details and advice can be derived. In the patient with adrenocortical insufficiency, any stressful event such as dental extraction requires extra hydrocortisone. Hydrocortisone 100 mg given

Chapter 11

orally 90 min (or parenterally 30 min) before any minor stressful event should suffice. If the stress is severe then up to 100 mg of hydrocortisone needs to be given by continuous intravenous infusion every 8 h until the patient has recovered.

Corticosteroid drugs

These are used as therapy for a variety of conditions:
1. Replacement therapy, e.g. Addison's disease, hypopituitarism, post-adrenalectomy,
2. Blood and lymphoid dyscrasias, e.g. thrombocytopenic purpura, aplastic anaemia, leukaemia, Hodgkin's disease,
3. Connective tissue diseases, e.g. giant cell (temporal) arteritis, systemic lupus erythematosus (SLE), polymyalgia rheumatica, systemic sclerosis and in some cases of rheumatoid arthritis,
4. Immunosuppression following organ transplantation,
5. Gut diseases, e.g. Crohn's disease, ulcerative colitis,
6. Allergic disorders, e.g. asthma, serum sickness,
7. Other uses, e.g. some renal diseases, chronic active hepatitis (hepatitis B negative), sarcoidosis,
8. Topical use, e.g. eczema, iridocyclitis.

Side-effects include:
(a) Muscle wasting,
(b) Diabetes mellitus,
(c) Osteoporosis,
(d) Salt and water retention and potassium loss; this results in oedema and hypertension,
(e) Suppression of local and general inflammatory responses thereby increasing the risk of infection, e.g. tuberculosis, opportunistic infections,
(f) Adrenocortical atrophy and impaired cortisol response to stress,
(g) Peptic ulceration or exacerbation of pre-existing ulcer symptoms,
(h) Cataract formation,
(i) Mental disturbances, e.g. psychosis,
(j) Appearance of Cushing's syndrome.

Types of corticosteroid. Prednisolone and prednisone (later converted to prednisolone in the liver) are the most widely used for the treatment of systemic diseases. Hydrocortisone is used for replacement therapy. Cortisone acetate is also used in replacement therapy but, as its absorption is less satisfactory than hydrocortisone, the latter is preferred by endocrinologists. Dexamethasone is used when high dosages are required with minimal salt and water retention (e.g. in reducing brain oedema). If aldosterone has to be replaced then fludrocortisone is used.

Common steroid preparations and their comparative strengths

1. Prednisolone	5 mg	4. Hydrocortisone	20 mg
2. Prednisone	5 mg	5. Dexamethasone	0.75 mg
3. Cortisone	25 mg	6. Triamcinolone	4 mg

Adrenal medulla
This part of the gland secretes adrenaline and noradrenaline. Both hormones are important in the maintenance of the blood pressure. An excess secretion (by a tumour of the adrenal medulla known as phaeochromocytoma) can produce profound hypertension often paroxysmal. Alpha (phenoxybenzamine) and beta (propranolol) adrenergic blocking drugs are used to control this condition prior to surgical removal of the tumour. Adrenaline is used therapeutically in the treatment of anaphylactic shock.

12 Diseases of bones and joints

ACQUIRED DISEASES OF BONES

Osteoporosis
Decreased amount of bone which is normal in composition.

Causes
The great majority of patients are women past the menopause in whom it is thought that lack of oestrogens leads to a gradual reduction in the bone mass.

In a small proportion of patients osteoporosis may result from immobilization, from endocrine disorders such as Cushing's syndrome, steroid treatment, hyperthyroidism or hypogonadism, or from malnutrition or malabsorption.

Clinical features
Loss of bone with age appears to be universal but only a minority of those affected have symptoms. The commoner symptoms are backache due to crush fractures of vertebrae, and fractures of long bones, particularly fractures of the neck of a femur or of a forearm. Fractures often result from slight trauma. The spinal fractures may lead to loss of height.

Even with appreciable bone loss conventional X-rays may show normal appearances, but deformity of vertebral bodies is often a helpful sign radiologically. The blood chemistry is usually normal.

Prevention
Immobilization should be avoided where possible in all patients. Progression of bone loss may be prevented in older women by replacement treatment with oestrogens. The indications for this

treatment are still controversial. A smaller reduction in the rate of bone loss can be achieved with calcium in some older patients.

Treatment
Established osteoporosis cannot be reversed, but in some patients further bone loss can be minimized by oestrogens or calcium. Fractures should be treated correctly with early mobilization where possible. In many patients with crush fractures of the vertebrae the pain from each episode lasts for one to two months.

Osteomalacia and rickets
Osteomalacia in adults and rickets in children are the diseases of bone caused by lack of vitamin D.

Causes
Since vitamin D is obtained either from the diet or from synthesis in the skin in the presence of ultraviolet radiation, deficiency does not occur unless a patient has both dietary deficiency and lack of exposure to sunshine. Those most at risk include house-bound elderly women and women, and children in Asian immigrant families.

Vitamin D deficiency can also result from gut diseases that cause malabsorption, particularly coeliac disease, pancreatic insufficiency and after partial gastrectomy.

Clinical features
Adults with osteomalacia complain of bone pains and muscle weakness. They may have a waddling gait and difficulty going up and down stairs. Clinical examination may show bone tenderness and fractures may occur.

In rickets bone pain is not always present. The major abnormality in the bone is in the epiphyses which are enlarged and radiologically abnormal. The epiphyseal changes may cause visible swelling, particularly in the distal parts of the radius and ulna, and at the junctions of the ribs with the costal cartilages (rickety rosary). If rickets remains untreated for a considerable period, bending of the long bones may occur giving either bow legs or knock knee. Dentition may be delayed.

Both in adults and in children vitamin D deficiency may cause hypocalcaemia sufficiently severe to cause tetany (Fig. 10), or carpopedal spasm.

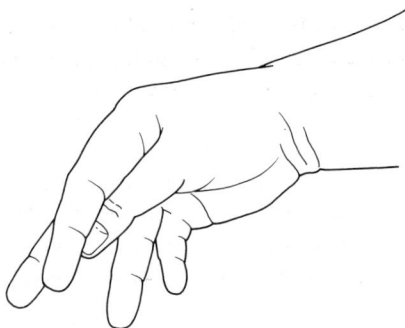

Fig. 10   'Main en graffe': a manifestation of hypocalcaemia.

Diagnosis
The diagnosis in adults depends on the serum chemistry; the serum calcium and serum inorganic phosphate levels are frequently low and the serum alkaline phosphatase is almost always raised. Serum levels of the vitamin D metabolite 25-hydroxyvitamin D are low. Radiology may reveal, in about a quarter of the patients, fracture-like translucencies known as pseudo-fractures.

In children the mainstay of diagnosis is radiology of the bone ends, particularly at the wrists and the knees.

Treatment
Vitamin D by mouth or with a single depot injection. Calcium supplements are thought to be helpful for the first two months of treatment.

Paget's disease of bone
This disorder is thought to be caused by a slow virus infection of osteoclasts. Affected bones are subject to repeated episodes of bone resorption by osteoclasts, followed by osteoblastic repair giving a very disorganized final structure with bone which though often radiologically dense, is soft, fragile and vascular.

Paget's disease affects approximately 3% of the British population aged over fifty. Some 90% of patients are asymptomatic. Those who do have symptoms may have pain in the affected bones or deformity. If the skull is involved it may increase in size, the patient may complain of headaches, and may suffer deafness. If the mandible or maxilla is affected progressive deformity may mean that dentures have to be replaced frequently. Bony ankylosis may link the teeth and the jaw.

Treatment
Only a minority of patients need treatment. The disorder may be suppressed with intramuscular injections of calcitonin or with the bisphosphonate drug disodium etidronate given by mouth.

Diagnosis
The radiological appearance of affected bones is characteristic. Serum calcium and phosphate levels are usually normal, but the serum alkaline phosphatase is raised and often very greatly raised.

Hyperparathyroidism
Excessive production of parathyroid hormone is most commonly caused by an adenoma of a single parathyroid gland. More rarely it results from carcinoma or from hyperplasia of usually all four glands.
   Secondary hyperparathyroidism is a term given to the increased parathyroid activity which occurs in response to hypocalcaemia, for example in renal failure or osteomalacia.

Clinical features
Many patients are asymptomatic and are discovered by chance as a result of biochemical screening. Patients may complain only of general symptoms such as weakness, malaise or tiredness but may, more characteristically, have constipation, excessive thirst, or form large quantities of urine (polyuria). Some patients present with renal colic due to the formation of renal stones. Others present with peptic ulceration; they occasionally have bone pain or fractures. Some of these patients may develop swellings in the bone; these may be found in the jaw and consist of osteoclasts or their remains (brown tumours).

Diagnosis
The serum calcium is raised and the serum phosphate is frequently low. The serum alkaline phosphatase is raised in about 5% of patients. Those more severely affected patients often have radiological abnormalities in the bones, notably subperiosteal erosions (best seen in the X-rays of the hands) and loss of the lamina dura. Cystic changes in the bones are only seen in the most severe cases.

Treatment
In most cases exploration of the neck leads to the surgical excision
of the parathyroid adenoma or carcinoma. Hyperplasia of the glands
requires removal of three of the glands and partial removal of the
fourth. Many elderly women with hyperparathyroidism, particularly
milder cases, require no treatment.

Other causes of hypercalcaemia
Hypercalcaemia frequently occurs as a result of malignant disease
either because of the bone metastases or because of the secretion by
the primary tumour of a substance with parathyroid hormone-like
actions. In some patients, even with advanced malignancy, treatment
of the hypercalcaemia may give worthwhile relief of symptoms.
Myeloma often causes hypercalcaemia.

Vitamin D Intoxication may result from therapeutic errors,
generally the administration of high-dose vitamin D preparations
(calciferol) in cases for whom it is not indicated, or in cases of
hypoparathyroidism who are not adequately followed up.

Hypoparathyroidism
Lack of parathyroid hormone with a resulting fall in serum clacium,
most commonly follows surgery in the neck in which the parathyroid
glands are removed or lose their blood supply. Rarely hypoparathyroidism may be congenital or result from an auto-immune disease.

Clinical features
Many patients with hypocalcaemia are irritable and some develop
convulsions. Tetany may occur (Fig. 10). If prolonged, hypoparathyroidism may lead to cataract formation. Untreated hypoparathyroidism
in childhood may lead to mental retardation.

Diagnosis
Serum calcium levels are always low, serum phosphate levels are
frequently high, alkaline phosphatase is normal. There are no reliable
radiological abnormalities.

Treatment
Acute episodes of tetany may be treated by slow intravenous injection
of calcium gluconate. In the longer term, patients are managed with
either vitamin D in large doses (calciferol) or with small doses of

alfacalcidol. Regular follow-up, with checks of the serum calcium level, is essential.

CONGENITAL DISEASES OF BONES

Osteogenesis imperfecta
This is a group of disorders of bone collagen all characterized by excessive fragility of the bones. In severe cases fractures may occur *in utero*. In milder cases the first fracture may not occur until the second or third year of life. Some of the more severely affected children die soon after birth or later in childhood, but many survive well into adult life. In the milder disease life expectancy is normal. About two thirds of the patients with osteogenesis imperfecta have a blue-grey discolouration of the sclerae. As with other disorders of collagen, joints may be hyperextensible. Some patients develop deafness which starts in the second or third decade of life. About half of the patients have discoloured fragile teeth due to dentinogenesis imperfecta.

Osteopetrosis
A very rare disorder, characterized by a great increase in bone density, it is also called 'marble bone disease' or 'Albers-Schönberg disease'. Some patients have a tendency to pathological fractures. Many patients become anaemic because of obliteration of the bone marrow.

Achondroplasia
An inborn abnormality inherited as a dominant, affecting those bones which develop from cartilage. Affected patients have short limbs but normal size trunks.

Fibrous dysplasia
This disorder (polyostotic fibrous dysplasia, McCune–Albright disease, Albright's disease) is a developmental disease but has no known genetic basis. Patients have pain and spontaneous fractures usually before the age of 10, and may have increasing deformity

thereafter. Radiographs of affected bones have a characteristic appearance with patches of rarefaction and sclerosis. The disease occurs most commonly in long bones but the skull or mandible may also be affected giving facial deformity. Some patients have skin pigmentation and precocious puberty.

Cleido-cranial dysplasia

This is a rare generalized bone dysplasia inherited as an autosomal dominant. Derformity of the skull is associated with disordered eruption of the teeth and long persistence of deciduous teeth. The most characteristic abnormality is the absence or small size of the clavicles so that the shoulder joints can be brought close to each other anteriorly.

DISEASES OF JOINTS

Osteoarthritis (osteoarthrosis or degenerative joint disease).

This is the most common joint disease. It affects all older people and especially heavy manual workers. As age advances there is progressive loss of cartilage from the bearing surface of weight-bearing and highly stressed joints. Eventually bone is exposed and ligaments become slack but to some extent stability is maintained by bony outgrowths or osteophytes at the joint margins. In the distal joints of the fingers, osteophytes are obvious behind the nails and are called Heberden's nodes. Other commonly affected joints are the hips, knees, great toes and spine, but any mechanically unsound joint can wear prematurely, e.g. malocclusion of the bite can lead to temporo-mandibular osteoarthritis.

Clinical features

The main symptoms are pain, stiffness, creaking on movement and, when the leg joints are affected, limping. Any joint swelling is bony hard and there is no evidence of inflammation such as warmth or soft tissue swelling as is seen in rheumatoid arthritis.

Diagnosis

Blood tests are normal so the diagnosis is confirmed by radiographs which show narrowing of the joint space and bony outgrowths (osteophytes).

Treatment
1. Aspirin or other drugs of anti-inflammatory analgesic type.
2. Weight reduction for the obese.
3. Eventually hips or knees may need surgical replacement with an artificial joint.

Rheumatoid arthritis

This disease of unknown aetiology affects about 2% of the population. It is most common in adults and especially females. The onset is gradual and the course fluctuating with exacerbations and remissions. While rheumatoid arthritis occasionally remits permanently, most patients develop deformity and disability after several years.

Inflammation first involves the synovial membrane and slowly extends on to the joint surface eroding cartilage, bone and ligaments. Other tissues may be affected causing pleurisy, pulmonary fibrosis, pericarditis, destruction of salivary and lacrimal glands and even inflammation of blood vessels which may lead to occlusion and gangrene.

Clinical features
The patient complains of pain, swelling and stiffness of joints which is worst on first rising and after resting. Several joints are affected, usually including those of the hands and feet. Involved joints are tender, warm, and feel spongy due to inflammation of the capsule and to fluid within the joint. The inflammation is not severe enough to cause redness of the overlying skin. Handgrips are weak and as articular surfaces are eroded away, deformities and restriction of movement develop. A Z-shaped thumb and ulnar deviation of the fingers due to subluxation (e.g. dislocation) at the metacarpo-phalangeal joints are very common.

Inflamed temporo-mandibular joints limit opening of the mouth. Damage to ligaments around the cervical spinal joints is a potential danger when procedures such as dental extraction are performed under general anaesthesia. Then, the voluntary muscles no longer splint the neck and sudden subluxation can crush the spinal cord causing paralysis.

Rheumatoid arthritis is rare in childhood, but when it occurs, inflammation of the temporo-mandibular joints causes premature fusion of the nearby epiphyses and a poorly developed mandible results. Orthodontic treatment is usually needed.

About 20% of patients develop rubbery, pea-sized subcutaneous nodules over bony prominences such as the elbows and knuckles. These occur especially in patients with extra-articular lesions such as vasculitis and Sjögren's syndrome.

Sjögren's syndrome is rheumatoid arthritis complicated by dry eyes and dry mouth from failing lacrimal and salivary secretions. The lack of flushing action leads to recurrent conjunctivitis and rapidly advancing dental caries.

Diagnosis
Investigation often reveals an accelerated blood sedimentation rate, a non-specific sign of inflammation, and a mild anaemia. The two most useful tests are X-rays which show erosion of articular surfaces, and the rheumatoid factor test. This antibody material is found in the blood of most patients which rheumatoid arthritis.

Treatment
General. Bed rest is rarely needed but heavy work aggravates inflammation so activities may need to be restricted. A night splint is often helpful for a painful large joint.

Drugs
1. *Non-steroidal anti-inflammatory drugs* such as aspirin, indomethacin and many others. These relieve mild pain but their anti-inflammatory action is minimal. Gastric irritation with ulceration and/or bleeding may occur. These drugs are adequate for mild rheumatoid arthritis causing pain but little joint damage.
2. *Second line drugs* such as *gold* injections (sodium aurothiomalate or myocrisin) and *penicillamine* may be added if pain is making life intolerable or if there is progressive joint damage. These drugs are unpredictable but about two thirds of patients respond over three months with gradual improvement. This can be maintained for long periods by continuous medication. Toxic reactions are common and either drug may need to be withdrawn because of rashes, mouth ulcers, renal damage or lack of blood platelets.
3. *Corticosteroids.* The most commonly used is prednisolone. If second line drugs fail or prove toxic, corticosteroids may be substituted. They damp down any inflammation but nowadays only small maintenance doses are used for side effects are frequent and dangerous with large doses, (p.148). Any rheumatoid patient with a florid round face is probably taking corticosteroids and

will carry a dosage card. After prolonged administration the small endogenous corticosteroid production is not required and the adrenal glands atrophy and can no longer boost production to deal with a stress such as a dental clearance. If a hypotensive collapse is to be avoided intra-muscular hydrocortisone should be given before the anaesthetic (p.298).

4. *Immuno-suppressive and cytotoxic drugs* such as azathioprine and cyclophosphamide. Although these drugs are mostly used to treat malignant disease, they do reduce the production of inflammatory cells and they are occasionally used to supplement corticosteroids in very severe rheumatoid arthritis and some other less common rheumatic diseases. They are important for they inhibit wound healing and they reduce resistance to infection. It is safer to stop these drugs for two or three weeks prior to surgery.

Surgery. The course of rheumatoid arthritis is punctuated by various surgical operations, e.g.

Removal of inflamed sheaths from the tendons around the wrists, preferably before tendon rupture has occurred,

Reshaping deformed feet to fit normal footwear,

Replacement of hip, knee and finger joints by artificial joints, i.e. arthroplasty.

Note. An inflammatory disease closely resembling rheumatoid arthritis occurs in some patients with psoriasis (p.264).

Ankylosing spondylitis

This chronic inflammatory disease of unknown aetiology starts in the sacro-iliac joints and slowly spreads in ascending fashion to involve the spinal joints; sometimes peripheral joints, especially the hips, knees and feet, are also affected. Although the early pathology resembles that of rheumatoid arthritis with erosion of joint surfaces by chronic inflammation, it differs later because the joint surfaces and nearby ligaments eventually fuse to become one bone.

Ankylosing spondylitis commonly affects young adults, especially males, and sometimes close relatives are affected. Most cell membranes carry antigens similar to those on red cells which are so important when blood is to be transfused. These tissue types are conveniently tested on leucocytes. There are many different human leucocyte antigens (HLA types) and one of these, B27, is found in approximately 5% of the general population and in 95% of ankylosing spondylitic patients. Why people with this tissue type are so susceptible to ankylosing spondylitis is not known.

Clinical features
The disease presents with backache and striking morning stiffness which causes difficulty with getting out of bed and with putting on stockings. Some patients also have attacks of inflammation of the iris of the eye (uveitis). In most cases the disease progresses up the spine and after a decade or more the pelvis, spine and ribs become one bone.

Diagnosis
The diagnosis is confirmed by an X-ray of the sacro-iliac joints, but if these are not clearly eroded it may be helpful to test for HLA B27.

Treatment
Physiotherapy. Since the spine will eventually fuse it is important to ensure that this occurs with an unbent position. Patients are advised to exercise each morning to strengthen the spinal extensor muscles which counteract any tendency to stoop.

Drugs. Pain is eased with non-steroidal anti-inflammatory drugs such as aspirin or indomethacin.

Note. Ankylosing spondylitis, Reiter's syndrome and psoriatic arthritis are related conditions and may coincide in the same patient or family.

Reiter's syndrome
This chronic polyarthritis mostly affects males and like ankylosing spondylitis it is much more common in patients with the B27 tissue type. It is a response to various infections remote from and not actually involving the joints and it is often called a reactive arthropathy. In the UK the most common trigger is non-specific urethritis (about 2% develop Reiter's syndrome) but it also follows various diarrhoeal illnesses including *B. flexner* dysentery.

Clinical features
A characteristic triad of arthritis, mostly affecting the leg joints, conjunctivitis and urethritis usually begins acutely but only the

arthritis persists for months or years. Mouth ulcers, inflammation of the glans penis and crusted pustule-like lesions on the soles of the feet may also occur.

Treatment
Although a course of tetracycline is given to the patient and his sexual partner this only clears the urethritis. The chronic arthritis is treated with non-steroidal anti-inflammatory drugs but severe attacks may require corticosteroids. Some patients develop ankylosing spondylitis and others develop peripheral joint deformities.

Gout
This is a metabolic disease. It commonly affects overweight, alcohol-drinking, middle-aged males. A few elderly females develop gout after prolonged treatment with diuretic drugs for heart failure or hypertension.

Cell nuclei from worn out body cells and from the nuclei of the more cellular protein foods are broken down to sodium monourate for excretion largely by the kidney. If urate production exceeds excretion, the body pool of urate increases. Being poorly soluble, urate precipitates in the joints, causing arthritis, and under the skin where it is visible as tophi. While many cases are due to an inherited metabolic abnormality leading to urate overproduction, other causes include increased cell breakdown, as in leukaemia, and inadequate urate excretion, due to kidney failure or to the excretion of urate blocking drugs such as diuretics and lactic acid produced from the metabolism of alcohol.

Clinical features
Attacks of gout are sudden, very painful, last a week or two and the first attack most often affects the first metatarso-phalangeal joint. The base of the great toe becomes hot, red, swollen and very tender. The attacks recur at intervals of weeks or months and as the urate pool increases, hard yellow tophi become visible in the helix of an ear and over bony prominences such as the point of the elbow.

Diagnosis
The diagnosis is confirmed by microscopic examination of synovial fluid for urate crystals and by the demonstration of a markedly raised level of urate in the blood.

Treatment
Diet. Weight reduction and the withdrawal of alcohol and urate-producing foods such as offal, meat extracts and dark flesh. Fish lowers the serum urate a little.

Two types of drug are always required:
Drugs to terminate the acute attack. These act by inhibiting the entrance of inflammation-producing cells into the affected joint. Although colchicine is effective it often causes diarrhoea, so maximal doses of a non-steroidal anti-inflammatory drug such as indomethacin are preferred and are given for a few days.

Drugs to reduce the body pool of urate. One of these drugs will be required for life. Allopurinol reduces urate production and is the least upsetting of these drugs. Probenecid increases renal excretion of urate but it sometimes causes dyspepsia.

Infective arthritis
In the UK only two joint infections occur with any frequency, viz. gonococcal and staphylococcal.

Gonococcal arthritis is seen especially in young adult females who are more likely than males to harbour the genital infection unknowingly long enough for waves of haematogenous spread to cause episodes of acute polyarthritis and septic skin lesions. There may be occasional mouth ulcers. The diagnosis is confirmed by cultures of blood, joint fluid, pustule contents and genital secretions. There is a rapid response to appropriate antibiotic treatment, but no longer are all gonococcal infections sensitive to penicillin.

Staphylococcal arthritis occurs in both sexes and tends to affect only one joint. The infection may originate from an unsterile intra-articular injection or from an infected boil or bunion with spread by the blood-stream or the lymphatics. The affected joint becomes painful, swollen, hot and maybe red over a period of several days. Antibiotic treatment needs to be continued for several weeks in order to kill organisms incarcerated in fibrino-purulent exudate.

13 Nutritional deficiency states and heavy metal poisoning

NUTRITIONAL DEFICIENCY STATES

Clinical observation, epidemiology and experimental work have defined separate clinical effects associated with deficiency of each nutrient. In clinical practice the situation is more complex in that even where the main problem is malnutrition, nutritional deficiencies are often multiple and associated with complications of malnutrition such as an increased susceptibility to infection.

In the UK nutritional deficiency is often the result of malabsorption so that the signs of deficiency are often combined with those of the underlying disease. The situation is even more complex in old age where subnutrition and multiple pathology often coexist. An example is that in old age glossitis is more likely to be due to poor oral hygiene, badly fitting dentures, a dry mouth, oral infections or heavy pipe smoking than to nutritional deficiency.

The following descriptions of nutritional deficiency, therefore, need to be interpreted with regard to the particular population under investigation.

Protein deficiency

Rich sources of animal protein include meat, fish and eggs. Sources of plant protein include legumes, bread and cereals. Although the amino acid proportions in animal and vegetable proteins are different, there is no evidence that animal proteins are of greater nutritional value than those of plants.

Protein deficiency is common in children in developing countries, but is also a problem in elderly people in the UK. The problem is exacerbated by conditions such as acute infections, trauma, surgery, chronic inflammation and malignancy. These increase catabolism, with protein breakdown, leading to negative nitrogen balance.

Features in adults include muscle wasting, a reduced resistance to infection, and in severe cases, hypoalbuminaemic oedema. Severe deficiency in children causes retarded growth, mental impairment, hypoalbuminaemia, oedema, and a reddish scaly depigmented skin (kwashiorkor).

Prevention should aim at educating mothers to increase the proportion of protein in the diet. If cereals and legumes are used this need not be too expensive. Correction of deficiency in the elderly is more difficult, but in extreme circumstances, high protein liquids given by nasogastric tube have been used with considerable benefit in frail elderly patients recovering from surgery.

Mineral deficiency

Iron

The richest sources of iron are red meat, heart, lung and kidney, but moderate quantities are contained in eggs, fish, whole wheat, oatmeal and leguminous vegetables. Deficiency may be due to a low intake, but more usual causes are malabsorption after gastric surgery or in coeliac disease, or excessive blood loss associated with menorrhagia, gastrointestinal disease or drugs such as salicylates damaging the gastric mucosa.

Deficiency causes dry brittle hair, vulvar pruritus and flattening or hollowing (koilonychia) of the nails. Many women with iron deficiency complain of tiredness, breathlessness, palpitations, dizziness and headaches, but these symptoms are equally common in women with normal iron status. More severe deficiency is associated with anaemia with all its attendant signs and symptoms (p.76).

Oral changes include soreness, atrophy and inflammation of the tongue (atrophic glossitis); cracking and redness of the corners of the mouth (angular stomatitis); and, occasionally, the formation of a band in the oropharynx (Plummer–Vinson or Patterson–Kelly syndrome) associated with dysphagia.

Deficiency is treated with ferrous sulphate tablets (p.78). More expensive preparations should only be used if the former cause a gastrointestinal upset.

Calcium

The main sources of calcium are milk, milk products and vegetables. Requirements are greatly increased during pregnancy. Severe deficiency is rarely a problem in the UK, but there is evidence that a marginally low intake increases the likelihood of osteoporosis (p.150) in old age. In childhood, dental development may also be compromised. The simplest way of correcting the problem is to increase the consumption of milk.

Skeletal decalcification and hypocalcaemia are usually the result of hypoparathyroidism (p.154) or vitamin D deficiency (p.166).

Potassium

High quantities of potassium are contained in meats, cereals, vegetables, fruits and fruit juices. Dietary deficiency of potassium can be a problem particularly in the elderly, but more common causes of depletion are diuretic therapy and severe diarrhoea.

The most serious consequence of potassium depletion is cardiac arrhythmia, particularly likely to occur if the patient is also on a cardiac glycoside. Other problems include muscle weakness, postural hypotension, carbohydrate intolerance, paralytic ileus and impaired renal concentrating ability.

Treatment is with potassium supplements such as effervescent potassium tablets or potassium in a slow-release matrix, but drinks such as tomato juice or orange juice contain high concentrations of potassium and are also useful. Patients requiring diuretics may be given potassium-sparing agents such as triamterene, amiloride or spironolactone.

Magnesium

Major sources of magnesium include bread, cereals, nuts and fruits, including bananas, avocados and dates. The signs and symptoms of magnesium deficiency are poorly recognized and often missed. They include anorexia, muscle weakness, tremor, ataxia, vertigo, depression, confusion, convulsions, tachycardia and cardiac arrhythmias, a list similar to that associated with chronic hypocalcaemia.

Treatment with magnesium salts poses problems in that these are osmotic laxatives and often cause diarrhoea. Bananas are particularly rich in magnesium and useful in mild deficiency.

Fluorine

Fluorine intake is determined mainly by its content in the local water supply. Deficiency increases the incidence and severity of dental caries. The most effective preventative measure is fluoridation of the water supply. Where political pressures prevent this, the use of toothpaste containing fluoride should be encouraged. Fluoride tablets have been used to control osteoporosis, but excessive doses cause skeletal decalcification so that the treatment remains controversial.

Iodine

The chief sources are drinking water, vegetables and fish. Since iodine is essential to the formation of the thyroid hormone, thyroxine, areas with a low intake are associated with a high incidence of goitre. This can be prevented by adding appropriate concentrations of iodide to table salt.

Vitamin deficiences

Fat-soluble vitamins

Vitamin A (retinol). This is available in food either as preformed retinol or as a precursor such as β-carotene which can be converted to retinol in the small bowel mucosa. Retinol is available only in butter, fortified margarine, eggs, milk, liver, fish and fish liver oils, but carotenoids occur in a wide range of green and yellow vegetables, e.g. spinach, cabbage, lettuce and carrots.

Signs of vitamin A deficiency include impairment of visual adaptation to dark, dryness and later keratinization of the cornea, and hyperkeratosis of the skin.

Oral changes consist of hyperplasia of the gums, and in infants, impaired dental development.

Deficiency can be prevented by giving 4000 units daily of vitamin A in halibut-liver oil capsules and growth deficiency states should be treated by a single high-dose tablet of the vitamin.

Vitamin D (calciferol). Vitamin D is present in low concentrations in butter, eggs and liver and in much higher concentrations in fish oils and fortified foods. The main source is cholecalciferol formed by the action of sunlight on cutaneous 7-dehydrocholesterol.

Deficiency results in skeletal decalcification. This presents in children as bowing of the long bones, stunted growth and deformity of the chest (rickets) (p.151). In young women osteomalacia (p.151) causes narrowing of the pelvic outlet with attendant obstetric problems. In the elderly osteomalacia increases the likelihood of fractures, particularly of the proximal femur. The vitamin deficiency also causes proximal muscle weakness so that patients have difficulty getting out of chairs and walk with a waddling gait. If the condition causes hypocalcaemia this produces irritability, anxiety, depression and latent or overt tetany.

In children, vitamin D deficiency may delay eruption of teeth. The condition can be treated with daily tablets of calcium and vitamin D.

Vitamin K. The main sources of vitamin K are green vegetables. It is essential to the formation of prothrombin so that deficiency produces a coagulation defect. Dietary deficiency is rare, but malabsorption due to liver disease, biliary disease or steatorrhoea frequently leads to prothrombin deficiency. This can be corrected by giving phytomenadione 10 mg daily orally or by injection. A single injection is used to correct bleeding due to overdosage of a coumarin anticoagulant. The vitamin is of no value where bleeding from a tooth socket is unrelated to a coagulation defect.

B complex vitamins

Thiamine (B_1). Sources of thiamine include cereals, yeast, eggs, pork and legumes. Milling cereals and cooking food at high temperatures reduces concentrations of thiamine. Deficiency may give rise to a high output cardiac failure (wet beri beri), a peripheral neuropathy (dry beri beri) or a smooth, sore tongue. Deficiency due to alcoholism causes mental impairment associated with ophthalmoplegia and ataxia (Wernicke's encephalopathy).

Since the condition is often assocated with other vitamin deficiencies it is commonly treated with a multi-vitamin preparation such as high potency Parentrovite by intravenous or intramuscular injection on alternate days for ten days. Less severe deficiency can be treated with a daily oral preparation, say, Orovite.

Riboflavine (B_2). Principal sources of riboflavine are yeast, milk, egg white, kidney, heart, liver and leafy vegetables.

Deficiency produces redness and inflammation of the lips (cheilosis), cracking of the angles of the lips (angular stomatitis) and redness, dryness, tenderness and atrophy of the tongue. Patchy denudation of papillae may produce the appearance of a 'geographical tongue'. Other effects of deficiency are seborrhoeic dermatitis, conjunctivitis and photophobia. Cataract and corneal opacity are uncommon complications. Treatment is as for thiamine deficiency.

Pyridoxine (B_6) deficiency has been implicated in causing a sore tongue as well as causing premenstrual symptoms. Although not proven, dietary supplementation with B_6 is prescribed commonly for these wide-ranging symptoms.

Niacin is a mixture including nicotinic acid, nicotinamide and their related compounds. These are present in cereals, but their bioavailability is dependent upon whether or not the niacin compounds can be hydrolysed. An example is that the niacin esters in maize cannot by hydrolysed so that clinical features of niacin deficiency are common in maize-eating parts of the world.

Non-infective glossitis is often the earliest symptom and may precede the skin lesions. There is a burning sensation or soreness in the mouth followed by angular stomatitis and cheilosis (a zone of red, denuded epithelium at the lip-closure line). The tongue has a characteristic scarlet, shiny, 'raw-beef' appearance caused by epithelial desquamation and because of oedema the tongue often shows indentations caused by the teeth.

The following are other features of niacin deficiency (pellagra):
1. Dermatitis, with hypersensitivity of exposed surfaces of the skin to light.
2. Diarrhoea.
3. Mental impairment, with anxiety and hallucinations.
Treatment is as for thiamine and riboflavine deficiency.

Folic acid. Sources of folic acid include green vegetables, yeast, liver and fruits, but the picture is complicated by the fact that there is considerable difference in the bioavailability of folic acid in different foodstuffs. It is also readily destroyed by heating.

Deficiency produces:
1. Megaloblastic anaemia.
2. Glossitis, and diarrhoea.
3. Mental impairment, spinal cord degeneration and a peripheral neuropathy.
Treatment is folic acid tablets.

Cyanocobalamin (B_{12}) deficiency is rarely the result of malnutrition but is usually the result of failure of the stomach to secrete intrinsic factor (*see* Pernicious anaemia, p.78). Here, too, the tongue may be smooth and sore.

Vitamin C (ascorbic acid)
The main sources of ascorbic acid are vegetables and fruit (particularly fruit juices). Heating destroys a large proportion of this in foodstuffs. Dietary deficiency is exacerbated by surgery, trauma and infections where metabolic requirements for vitamin C are increased.

Severe deficiency produces the clinical picture of scurvy:
1. Gingivitis with sponginess and bleeding of the gums, foetid breath, and loosening of teeth,
2. Anaemia,
3. Perifollicular skin haemorrhages, subcutaneous sheet haemorrhages, and gastrointestinal bleeding,
4. Apathy, weakness, lethargy and depression,
5. Subperiosteal haemorrhage with bone pain (in children),
6. Failure of wound healing.

In less severe forms its effect, particularly in the elderly, is to delay the healing of traumatic and surgical wounds, varicose ulcers and pressure areas.

Treatment is with oral ascorbic acid tablets.

HEAVY METAL POISONING

With improved hygiene in industry, gross heavy metal poisoning is rare but a wide variety of metal compounds and metalloids can affect the mouth and throat and a careful occupational history must always be taken in patients with non-infective conditions.

Lead

Lead ingested or inhaled as fumes continues to be a problem, although mainly in small industries where the dangers are not recognized.

Children may become poisoned by chewing lead or lead-painted objects. The symptoms are:

Metallic taste in the mouth,
Weakness,
Colicky abdominal pain,
Anaemia.

In the long-term there may be peripheral neuropathy and CNS effects. A blue line on the gums is rare and is only found in the presence of caries.

Mercury

Mercury is still widely used in the chemical industry and cases of domestic poisoning are still reported from mercury spillage in the home. Dentistry carries a special risk from the preparation of amalgams. Mercury vaporizes easily and a small rise in temperature greatly increases vapour pressure. Smoking is an important risk factor because mercury may be transferred from the hands on to the cigarette and vapourized at the elevated temperatures. Erythema of the hands (pink disease) is commoner in children but may also be seen in adults. Chronic poisoning may be associated with headache, irritability, insomnia, fatigue, muscle and joint pains and timidity. Later muscular tremors and incoordination may develop, which may be confused with alcoholism. The patient may complain of a metallic taste and excessive salivation. There may be an associated stomatitis and pharyngitis. Urinary mercury levels are often a poor guide to poisoning and it is helpful to have nail and hair samples analysed as a measure of the body's mercury burden. None of these methods provide a reliable indication of the amount of mercury in the central nervous system.

Treatment with chelating agents is remarkably effective and the neurological abnormalities usually subside.

It is most important to thoroughly remove all mercury from working surfaces and clean meticulously after any spillage.

14 Neurological disorders

MOTOR FUNCTION AND NEUROLOGICAL DISORDERS

Impairment of posture and movement arises from disorders affecting many sites in the nervous system: the upper motor neurone, the cerebellum, the extrapyramidal motor system, lower motor neurone, the neuromuscular junction and muscles. These produce a variety of disorders of movement of the facial muscles, the jaw, pharynx, palate, tongue, and the neck, as well as the trunk and limbs. The motor system is illustrated in Fig. 11.

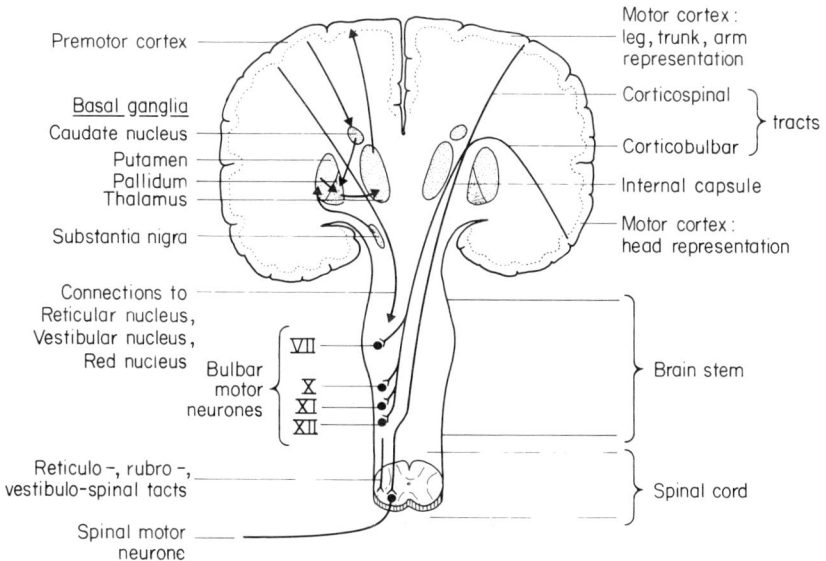

Fig. 11 Motor pathways.

Upper motor neurone

Descending corticobulbar and corticospinal pathways arise from the motor cortex in a topographical representation of the body, the homunculus. Closely associated with these pathways are descending extrapyramidal fibres from the adjacent premotor cortex. These pathways descend through the internal capsule; the corticobulbar pathway terminates in the brainstem while the corticospinal pathways cross at the pyramids and descend in the lateral columns of the spinal cord to terminate in synapses at the anterior horn cells.

Several common disorders affect these pathways.

Stroke. This term covers both cerebral infarction and haemorrhage. Infarction may be caused by embolism from the heart or great vessels, thrombosis of cerebral vessels, or reduction of cerebral perfusion. Cerebral haemorrhage includes bleeding from large (berry) aneurysms and arteriovenous malformations, and from small microaneurysms which are common in hypertension. Haemorrhage may also occur in patients with a bleeding tendency or after trauma as intracerebral, subdural or extradural haemorrhage. Stroke is commoner in the elderly, and especially with a history of hypertension, diabetes, cardiac or blood disorders. About one-third of patients who suffer from acute strokes die, one-third make a complete recovery, and one-third have persistent neurological deficits. Some patients have transient neurological disorders lasting for less than 24 hours, called transient ischaemic attacks.

Multiple sclerosis results from zones of demyelination of myelinated pathways in the central nervous system. Therefore, motor disorder may arise from lesions in the corticobulbar and corticospinal tracts, the cerebellum or brainstem. Sensory, visual, bladder and mental symptoms also may develop. Younger patients may have a slowly progressing weakness of limbs. These symptoms may be exacerbated by infection, fatigue, change in temperature. Anaesthesia is not precluded.

Congenital spastic disorders. These affect corticospinal and corticobulbar pathways, but some patients also have an extrapyramidal and/or cerebellar involvement.

Cerebral tumours. These are primary tumours (glioma, meningioma) or metastatic tumours (commonly from the lung or breast).

Cerebral degenerations. Mental impairment is often greater than weakness, e.g. memory impairment in Alzheimer's disease is the dominant feature, and bilateral weakness usually occurs late in the progressive deterioration.

Motor neurone diseases (*see* p.177).

Metabolic diseases. This includes effects of alcohol and vitamin B_{12} deficiency.

Infections (severe meningitis, encephalitis, cerebral abscess).

Clinical features

Unilateral lesions. Except for the lower part of the face, the bulbar muscles have bilateral innervation and therefore tend to be little affected by unilateral upper motor neurone pathology. Thus in a patient with hemiparesis from a stroke, mild or moderate impairment of movement of the lower part of the face may occur. Closure of the eye is sometimes affected in severe acute lesions, but movement of the frontalis in frowning or wrinkling the forehead is unimpaired. Voluntary movement is more impaired than involuntary. Thus a patient may not be able to show teeth on request but may have greater movement automatically in smiling or laughing.

Bilateral lesions—pseudobulbar palsy. In contrast to the mild deficits of unilateral lesions, severe problems arise with bilateral upper motor neurone lesions. *Dysarthria* (impaired articulation) occurs because of reduced movement of the facial muscles, the soft palate, pharynx and larynx. If the laryngeal muscles are affected the voice volume may be reduced with difficulty in phonating (*dysphonia*). The laryngeal defect may also cause difficulty in clearing secretions and predispose to chest infections. Swallowing is impaired but the gag reflex remains. The tongue cannot be protruded. In severe cases, patients cannot speak (*anarthria*) or swallow (*aphagia*).

Cerebellum
Cerebellar signs arise from lesions either in the hemisphere or in the midline structures (vermis). The cerebellum is linked by afferent and efferent connections with important brainstem nuclei: vestibular, olivary, red nuclei, the cuneatus and gracilis nuclei, the reticular formation and thalamus.

Causes of cerebellar disorders
Disorders that affect the cerebellum include intoxication with alcohol and phenytoin (p.182), strokes, tumour, multiple sclerosis and degenerations that specifically affect the cerebellum and its connections, e.g. Friedreich's ataxia or idiopathic cerebellar degeneration.

Clinical features
Lesions of the cerebellum impair the performance of complex coordinated voluntary movements without causing weakness. In the limbs this inaccuracy can be seen during movement so that smooth movement is broken up, particularly at the end of intended movement (*intention tremor*), the movement is clumsy and the walking unsteady. A unilateral lesion affects the ipsilateral side. In a midline (vermis) lesion there may be little or no limb ataxia, but the patient is very unsteady when standing or sitting (*truncal ataxia*). Movement of bulbar muscles is affected in bilateral lesions producing slurred, indistinct speech. The normal cadence and rhythm of speech may be replaced by more laboured, slow speech with emphasis on each syllable. The more automatic movements of swallowing are unimpaired. Jerking eye movements (*nystagmus*) occur.

Extrapyramidal system
The extrapyramidal system is a complex group of interconnected nuclei concerned with posture and movement. The major components are the substantia nigra, the caudate nucleus, putamen, pallidum and thalamus, with connections to the cortex, brainstem and cerebellum.

Parkinson's disease
The commonest extrapyramidal disorder is Parkinson's disease caused by gradually developing loss of dopamine-containing cells in the basal ganglia. It usually develops over the age of 50 years. There are three clinical problems. The first is tremor, which usually starts in the limbs but may spread to involve the head and jaw. A prominent head or jaw tremor makes fitting of dentures difficult. The second component is rigidity which is an increased resistance of muscles to movement in the affected limbs. Patients become increasingly flexed, including the neck. The third component is hypokinesis (or bradykinesis), a slowness in movement with difficulty in initiating or changing patterns of movement. Starting and stopping walking, turning and using the hands are difficult. Speech may become unclear

and of low volume. Saliva may be cleared slowly, with dribbling from the mouth (*drooling*). Some patients have difficulty in swallowing (*dysphagia*).

Other extrapyramidal disorders

In *orofacial dyskinesias* continuous smacking movements of the lips, face and tongue occur, usually following long-term phenothiazine and butyrophenone therapy (tardive dyskinesias).

In *chorea* similar movements occur in the face, but there are also quick semi-purposive movements of the arms and legs.

Dystonia is a focal fixed posture. This includes torticollis in which there is embarrassing and usually painful twisting of the head to one side, and rarely dystonia of the jaw and facial muscles.

Myoclonus is a sudden jerking of muscles found in some patients with epilepsy, but also in other neurological disorders. They may involve the face as well as the limbs.

In *athetosis* there is slow writhing movement of the limbs, and in *hemiballismus* there is wild flailing movement of the limbs on one side.

LOWER MOTOR NEURONES

These arise in the brainstem and in the anterior horns of the spinal cord to supply voluntary muscles. Large fibres (alpha efferents) innervate skeletal muscle, and small fibres (gamma efferents) innervate muscle spindles which are involved in the control of muscle tone. The motor neurones are activated by descending corticobulbar and corticospinal connections and also by monosynaptic and polysynaptic reflex pathways at the spinal level. Lesions of the motor neurones, their axons or myelin sheaths result in weakness and wasting of muscle and spontaneous contractions or twitching of superficial muscle (fasciculation).

The facial nerve arises in the pons (where it can be damaged by stroke, multiple sclerosis, etc.). It passes with the acoustic and vestibular nerves through the internal auditory canal, and is vulnerable to compression by an acoustic nerve tumour. The ganglion may be damaged in geniculate herpes in which pain develops together with vesicles on the tongue, palate and ear. The nerve traverses the petrous-temporal bone, where it is liable to damage in base of skull fractures or middle ear infection. It emerges at the stylomastoid foramen, the probable site of the lesion in idiopathic Bell's palsy, to pass through the parotid gland to the muscles of the face. Taste over the anterior two-thirds of the tongue is supplied via the chorda tympani branch.

In Bell's palsy facial paralysis develops rapidly over several hours, and may last for weeks or months. The facial palsy usually affects all muscle groups and the patient cannot smile, pout, close the eye or wrinkle the forehead. Speech is impaired. The most important early problem is drying of the cornea and complicating infection. With partial reinnervation regrowth of the nerve fibres may be abberent so that, for example, an attempt at smiling may produce a wink. A small proportion of patients fail to recover and may become disturbed by the cosmetic effects of facial palsy. The early treatment is steroids and the prevention of damage to the eye.

The trigeminal nerve is predominantly sensory to the face and much of the scalp, but the motor component is distributed with the mandibular branch to innervate the temporalis, masseter, pterygoids and other small muscles in the neck. Bilateral weakness impairs chewing. The jaw deviates to the affected side in a unilateral lesion. The trigeminal nerve is affected in stroke, multiple sclerosis, tumour, shingles and trigeminal neuralgia.

The vagus (10th) nerve is motor to the palate, the pharynx, the upper oesophagus and the larynx as well as supplying the parasympathetic fibres to the heart, lungs and upper gut. Palatal palsy results in the nasal escape of air during speech, and regurgitation of fluids through the nose on swallowing. Pharyngeal palsy impairs swallowing and speech. Laryngeal palsy produces dysphonia. Respiratory secretions are difficult to clear. This is particularly important for anaesthetic procedures. The gag reflex is impaired. This is elicited by touch of the posterior pharyngeal wall (via the glossopharyngeal nerve); the pharynx and palate then contract.

The accessory (11th) nerve innervates the sternomastoid and upper part of the trapezius muscles. Weakness of the left sternomastoid results in weakness in looking to the right (and vice versa). Bilateral weakness results in weakness in thrusting the head forward. The trapezius muscle elevates the shoulder. Lesions of the accessory nerve usually arise with complex intrinsic brainstem lesions or rarely from pressure on the nerve from tumours as they emerge from the posterior fossa, e.g. glomus jugulare tumour.

Hypoglossal (12th) nerve innervates the tongue. Lesions occur occasionally in isolation (possibly post-viral), in medullary lesions or from nerve compression with rare tumours. Unilateral lesions produce a wasted half of the tongue that is poorly protruded and deviates to the side of the lesion. Fasciculation is best seen with the tongue lying at rest in the floor of the mouth, for maintained protrusion produces tongue movements which may be difficult to distinguish from fasciculation.

Bulbar palsies

Bulbar palsies produce severe disorder with dysarthria, dysphonia, dysphagia and nasal regurgitation, but differ from bilateral upper motor neurone lesions (pseudobulbar palsy). These most frequently arise from:

1. Motor neurone disease, a rare, grim neurological disorder with progressively increasing upper and lower motor neurone lesions;
2. Polio, fortunately now rare in Europe and the USA because of immunization;
3. The Gullain–Barré syndrome, an uncommon severe demyelinating disorder of peripheral nerves producing weakness of the limbs also;
4. Rare extension of inflammatory disorders to the cranial nerves in sarcoidosis and tuberculosis.

Neuromuscular junction

Transmission from nerve to muscles is by acetylcholine. In myasthenia gravis cholinergic receptors are damaged by circulating antibodies, impairing this transmission. Patients therefore fatigue unduly easily. Ocular muscles only may be affected, but bulbar muscle weakness can be an important feature. Patients often describe fatigue during chewing, and that the voice volume diminishes and the speech slurs during conversation. These patients are vulnerable to a variety of drugs, including some antibiotics, analgesics and neuromuscular blocking agents. Therefore, *meticulous care is needed in the management of myasthenic patients and procedures requiring anaesthesia should be done in hospital.*

Muscle disorders

Muscles are affected by inflammatory diseases (polymyositis), drugs, metabolic and endocrine disease, and in inherited dystrophies. The

main effects are trunk and limb weakness. Bulbar muscles are involved only in very severe myopathies, e.g. dysphagia may occur in
severe polymyositis. *In facioscapulohumeral dystrophy* facial muscle
weakness may restrict smiling, and eye closure; the facial muscles
sag, the mouth may hang open, and the sternomastoid and trapezius
muscles become thin; proximal muscles of the limbs are also weak.
In *myotonic dystrophy* a characteristic facial appearance is seen with
prefrontal balding, ptosis, facial weakness, wasting of the masseters,
temporalis and sternomastoid muscles, as well as limb muscles.
Impaired swallowing may occur. The term myotonia describes an
inability to relax after voluntary contraction, usually seen in the
limbs, but it can be demonstrated in the tongue and facial muscles. A
cardiomyopathy may occur with heart failure and arrhythmias indicating a need for *special care with anaesthesia.*

Fits, faints and funny turns
Episodes of coma, altered consciousness, or odd behaviour may arise
from impaired blood flow to the brain (syncope), epilepsy, metabolic
changes such as hypoglycaemia and drugs, or mental disorder.

Syncope
Syncope commonly arises from fear and stress with reduced cardiac
output and constriction of skin vessels. It may also be secondary
to cardiac arrhythmia, severe haemorrhage, postural hypotension,
particularly after drugs, after coughing, and rarely when pressure on
an abnormally sensitive carotid sinus induces reflex cardiac slowing.
    The patient may have prodromal symptoms of darkening vision,
nausea, a sense of rotation, lightheadedness or muzziness, and the
patient is seen to become pale, sweaty, confused or unconscious.
The muscles become flaccid. Treated properly, the patient usually
recovers rapidly (p.49). A seizure may complicate a prolonged
syncope and is an indication of severe syncope and not of epilepsy.

Treatment. The patient should be lain flat, on the side, in the coma
position, the airway cleared and allowed to recover. Prolonged coma
requires urgent hospital treatment.

Transient ischaemic attacks
These are episodes of neurological dysfunction lasting for less than 24
hours, commonly for minutes only, arising from a vascular cause. They

occur most commonly in older patients, especially with a history of hypertension and diabetes. They may be caused by emboli arising from the heart, aorta, or extracranial vessels which lodge in the cerebral circulation. They may also be triggered by a reduction in cardiac output with cardiac arrhythmia or myocardial infarct, or sometimes with kinking of the carotid or vertebral arteries in the neck when turning the head. Transient hemiplegia, hemianaesthesia, impairment of language (dysphasia), vertigo, diplopia, or incoordination may occur. Patients should be referred for further investigation. The choice of treatments include aspirin for reducing platelet aggregation, anticoagulants (usually for cardiac emboli), and surgery for extracranial atheroma.

Hypoglycaemia
Hypoglycaemia may arise in diabetics with excessive insulin or inadequate food, in patients with previous gastric surgery and occasionally other patients. Clinical features are altered perception, confusion, agitation, occasionally aggression, or coma. The patient is often sweaty. Convulsions may occur.

Treatment is with oral glucose in the early stage, but if the patient loses consciousness, with intravenous glucose.

Panic attacks/hyperventilation
Some fearful patients develop a sense of panic or fear, they breathe rapidly and shallowly and complain of paraesthesiae in the limbs and face. Severe cases may have carpopedal spasm and loss of consciousness. The treatment is to allay anxiety in the early stage, if possible, or to get the patient to rebreathe into a bag.

Hysteria
Bizarre behaviour, including loss of consciousness, may arise from a psychological cause, and the differentiation from other diseases is based on careful analysis of the events preceding the attack, the behaviour during the episode, and the patient's personality.

Further investigations may be needed.

Epilepsy
Epilepsy is a common disorder with a prevalence of 1 in 200 people having had recent seizures or receiving an anticonvulsant. Many people have a single seizure triggered by syncope, drug or alcohol withdrawal, and only when seizures are recurrent is the diagnosis

of epilepsy made. Epilepsy is commonest in childhood and young adults, but may occur at any age.

There are several types of seizures:

Generalized—arising from bilateral cerebral discharges.
1. *Tonic-clonic seizures (grand mal).* A dramatic seizure starts with a sudden cry, loss of consciousness, intense generalized (tonic) muscle contraction so that the limbs often become extended and the back arched. As breathing ceases the patient becomes blue. The eyes are often deviated upwards. Then, infrequently at first, the patient begins to jerk (the clonic phase) and the tongue may be bitten by the clonic movements of the jaws. The jerking gradually settles to leave the patient in coma. Incontinence may occur. The patient gradually recovers over several minutes and is often confused initially, occasionally with odd behaviour (post-ictal automatism) or with vomiting, headache, drowsiness or aching limbs.
2. *Absence seizures (petit mal).* Absence attacks last for seconds with a brief interruption in consciousness, sometimes accompanied by eyelid flickering. In prolonged attacks fumbling hand movements or movements of the face may occur. Absence attacks may occur very frequently, up to hundreds of times a day. They are most common in childhood.
3. *Myoclonus.* This is a sudden jerk of muscles, either bilaterally or unilaterally. It occurs in epilepsy, but may arise also with other diseases that affect the cortex, brainstem or spinal cord.

Partial seizures arise from focal lesions in the cerebral cortex. The site of the lesion determines the type of fit. A lesion in the motor cortex produces twitching movements of a limb on the opposite side. A sensory cortex lesion produces localized sensory symptoms on the contralateral side. An occipital focus may produce contralateral unformed visual hallucination. The commonest partial seizures, however, arise from discharge in the temporal lobes, the adjacent frontal cortex and deeper limbic structures, causing *temporal lobe epilepsy*. A variety of symptoms and signs occur. The patient may describe an odd, ill-defined rising sensation from the epigastrium to the head; dizziness; complex perceptual changes with the environment looking very familiar (déja vu) or oddly different (jamais vu), very large, small or distant. There may be hallucinations of smell, intense fear or anger. The patient may lose consciousness and do complex inappropriate activity (automatism) of which there is no subsequent recollection. Often the patient simply remains 'cut-off', inactive, and seemingly in a dream state. Occasionally there may be running or laughing.

Partial seizures may spread to become generalized tonic-clonic seizures.

Status epilepticus. Status epilepticus is recurrent seizures without regaining consciousness. It is a medical emergency.

Management of epilepsy

Treatment of a tonic-clonic seizure. The seizure cannot be terminated, and the aim is to prevent injury. The patient should be removed from nearby dangers and lain flat. Tight clothing should be loosened. Do not attempt to insert a gag between clenched teeth for this may produce dental trauma. Suffocation can occur during a seizure from the tongue falling back and obstructing the pharynx or from a broken denture in the throat. When the tonic-clonic phase settles, the patient should be placed on a side, with the head tilted down, loose dentures removed, and the airway cleared. If status epilepticus is present, treatment is with intravenous diazepam (p.183) and transfer to intensive medical care. The emulsion of diazepam (Diazemuls) should be used as otherwise intravenous diazepam carries the danger of thrombophlebitis.

Prevention of seizures

General measures. The patients should avoid triggers such as excessive alcohol, stress or fatigue. Driving is precluded until a patient has been fit-free for two years except for HGV and PSV licences for which patients have to be fit-free from the age of five years. Other advice depends on the patient's job and recreations. Dangerous jobs are precluded. Swimming is precluded in patients with uncontrolled seizures unless supervised. Patients with uncontrolled seizures are advised to avoid deep baths, and those with sleep seizures should avoid pillows unless of safety type.

Anticonvulsants. The aim of treatment with anticonvulsant drugs is to suppress fits by maintaining an effective concentration of the drug in the plasma, and hence in the brain. The dose and frequency of administration of the drug are influenced by its plasma half-life. With most anti-epileptic drugs twice daily dosage is satisfactory; when large doses are required it is sometimes better for the drug to be taken three or four times daily. Careful adjustment of dosage is necessary, gradually increasing until the fits are controlled or toxicity limits further increase in dosage. With some anti-epileptic drugs, plasma levels can be measured and the dosage adjusted to maintain the level in the therapeutic range. Whenever possible, patients should be treated regularly with a single anticonvulsant drug, in optimum dosage. A second drug is added only if toxic effects limit adequate dosage or if fits continue despite high doses of the first drug. Once a satisfactory therapeutic regime is established it should be continued until there is freedom from fits for at least 2–3 years. Anticonvulsant therapy should never be stopped abruptly as this may precipitate a series of convulsions (status epilepticus). Anaesthetists should be warned about anticonvulsant drugs being taken by the patient as this may influence the anaesthetic management. If seizures of various types occur in the same person, additional treatment with other anticonvulsants may be necessary. *Phenytoin, sodium valproate*, and *carbamazepine* are similarly effective for the treatment of tonic-clonic and partial seizures. *Phenobarbitone* and *primidone* are widely used but less satisfactory because of prominent sedation and behavioural effects in children. *Sodium valproate* or *ethosuximide* is used for absence attacks (petit mal). Sodium valproate or *clonazepam* is used for myoclonus.

Phenytoin is a good anticonvulsant, effective in controlling grand mal epilepsy. *Gingival hyperplasia* occurs in 10–25% of patients. It is worse with higher doses and prolonged treatment. It is also more prominent anteriorly than posteriorly and on the buccal and labial surfaces of the teeth than the lingual. It is associated with poor dental hygiene and low IgA concentrations in saliva. In mildly affected patients attention to dental hygiene may prevent worsening. In severe cases alternative anticonvulsants should be considered. If there are no alternatives, surgical procedures for the hyperplasia should be considered.

Coarsening of facial features, acne and hirsutism are additional adverse cosmetic effects of chronic usage, particularly in younger patients. Acute neurological effects include nausea, drowsiness, ataxia, and nystagmus at high doses, but subtle slowing of function may occur even with blood levels in the optimal range for controlling seizures. The drug thus has a narrow therapeutic index and it is usual to control the dose by monitoring its plasma concentration. Rare adverse effects are hepatotoxicity, folate deficiency (which may cause megaloblastic anaemia, p.78, that responds to folic acid therapy) osteomalacia and immune abnormalities.

Carbamazepine is also effective in controlling grand mal epilepsy and is the drug of choice for partial seizures. It is less sedative than phenytoin but dosage is sometimes limited by adverse effects which include drowsiness, dizziness, ataxia and diplopia. Skin rashes may occur.

Sodium valproate is a newer but generally well-tolerated drug effective in controlling grand mal seizures but it may produce mild alopecia, tremor, weight gain, and drowsiness. Rare fatal hepato-toxicity and pancreatitis have been described. Its relative value compared to carbamazepine and phenytoin is still being assessed.

Barbiturates such as phenobarbitone and primidone (which is partly converted to phenobarbitone in the body) may be well-tolerated, but the commonest adverse effects are sedation and hyperactivity in children. Their use has declined.

Diazepam is the treatment of choice for status epilepticus, given in adults in an initial 10 mg i.v. bolus. It is not useful as a long-term anticonvulsant.

Clonazepam is effective in status epilepticus, and may be given as an oral anticonvulsant. The main adverse effect is sedation.

Headache

The diagnosis of headache and facial pain requires a careful history of the site and type of pain, factors which trigger or exacerbate the pain, and factors which may relieve the pain. Other symptoms such as nausea, vomiting, visual symptoms, nasal stuffiness, lacrimation, may help in the assessment. Frontal sinusitis and ocular pain have to be distinguished from other causes of headache. Dental pain may be referred to the maxillary, temporal and frontal regions and the following disorders may be diagnostic or management problems.

Migraine

Migraine is common, affecting about 10% of women and 5% of men, mainly in the first three decades. It arises from complex changes in both the extracranial and the intracranial vessels, usually with an initial phase of vasoconstriction, followed by a phase of vasodila-tation. It may be triggered by a variety of stimuli: fasting, anxiety, menstruation, exertion, foods, e.g. coffee, chocolate, cheese, red wines.

The throbbing unilateral headache may be located behind the eye, in the forehead, or temple. It may, however, spread to the entire half of the scalp (hemicrania) or bilaterally. Although usually throbbing, it is sometimes perceived as a tight pain. Nausea, and sometimes vomiting, occur and the patient prefers to lie in a darkened room. Sleep may be helpful.

In classical migraine there are features of cerebral cortical dysfunction preceding the headache phase by 10–30 minutes. These are frequently visual symptoms, e.g. complex patterns of flashing or zig zag lights, or loss of vision. Rarely hemianopia, hemiparesis or complex changes in the patient's perception of the environment may occur.

The management is to avoid the precipitants, if possible. Simple analgesics should be used, e.g. aspirin or paracetamol, taken at the start of the headaches. Some proprietary preparations of aspirin or paracetamol include metoclopramide to reduce the nausea and increase the rate of absorption of the analgesic. Ergotamine-containing preparations may be used in patients who do not respond to analgesics. Ergotamine relieves migraine by constricting cranial arteries but visual and other prodromal symptoms are not helped and vomiting may be made worse. Repeated administration of ergotamine preparations may cause habituation and chronic overdosage may, rarely, provoke headache.

Prophylactic drugs, e.g. pizotifen or propranolol, may be used for refractory, frequent migraine. Pizotifen is an antihistamine and antiserotonergic drug, related to the tricyclic antidepressants, whereas propranolol is a β-adrenoceptor blocking drug which may dilate constricted cerebral vessels but prevent dilatation of the extracranial vessels.

Migrainous neuralgia (cluster headache). Although migrainous neuralgia is caused also by complex vascular changes, the clinical features are distinct from migraine. The pain may be located behind the eye, or in the maxillary region (lower half headache), and is an agonizing throbbing pain lasting for 30 minutes to 3 hours, recurring in bouts of one or more daily for several days or weeks before remitting for weeks, months or years. It occurs almost entirely in men, and may waken the patient from sleep. Lacrimation, rhinorrhoea, or erythema of the skin in the affected area may occur but vomiting is not a feature. In contrast to migraine, the patient does not find comfort in lying quietly.

Drug treatment includes ergotamine, pizotifen, indomethacin (an anti-inflammatory, analgesic drug) and lithium. The diverse mode of action of these drugs reflects the complex and poorly understood nature of the disorder.

Atypical facial pain. This is a dull, continuous pain in the maxillary region lasting for days or weeks, usually in middle-aged women with some features of depression. There are no physical signs.

The treatment is with antidepressants.

Tension headache (muscle contraction headache). This is commonly a dull discomfort in the frontal and/or occipital regions. The pain may also be described as pressure on the vertex, a tight band around the head, or there may be localized scalp tenderness. It may be clearly associated with stress, but some patients develop chronic persistent pain in which the initial trigger is difficult to identify. The treatment is with simple analgesics and discussion of the source of stress.

Temporal arteritis. This is a disease of the elderly, often accompanied by malaise and fatigue. The pain may be mild or severe, located in the temporal region, but sometimes also in the occipital region, face or jaw. The erythrocyte sedimentation rate (ESR) is high, and temporal artery biopsy may show characteristic vasculitic changes. Urgent treatment is required with steroids because of the risk of blindness from ischaemic optic neuropathy.

Shingles
Shingles are caused by the herpes-zoster virus invading dorsal roots including the trigeminal nerve. Pain may present a diagnostic problem in the early stage as it precedes a crop of small fluid-filled vesicles by a few days. The development of the vesicles usually makes the diagnosis clear. These vesicles crust then heal leaving slightly scarred skin. The greatest early risk is a lesion of the cornea. In about 10% of patients pain persists for weeks, months or even years, as *post-herpetic neuralgia.* This is a persistent, dull, gnawing, debilitating pain, commonly affecting sleep, and results in understandable secondary depression. It may be partially alleviated by analgesics, tricyclic drugs, e.g. amitriptyline and/or by carbamazepine if there is a paroxysmal component to the pain.

Trigeminal neuralgia

The cause of trigeminal neuralgia is unclear but there is now evidence to suggest arterial compression of the trigeminal nerve as it enters the brainstem. It usually develops over the age of 60. In some younger patients there may be other structural diseases, e.g. multiple sclerosis. Patients describe bouts of intense sharp pain most commonly in the mandibular division, occasionally also in the maxillary division but rarely in the ophthalmic division. The bouts of pain last for seconds or sometimes minutes, and may be triggered by eating, speaking, touch, or cold winds. At their worst, patients do not wish to talk, eat, wash, shave or move.

The treatment of choice is carbamazepine which is effective in 70–80%. Some patients have a spontaneous remission. Thermocoagulation of the trigeminal nerve or other surgical procedures may be required in refractory patients.

Glossopharyngeal neuralgia

In this rare disorder there are paroxysmal bouts of pain in the palate and neck, similar in quality to trigeminal neuralgia. The treatment of choice is also carbamazepine.

Tumour

Intracranial tumours produce pain only with increased intracranial pressure, direct involvement of cranial nerves, e.g. trigeminal, or damage to meninges or large arteries. The headache of increased intracranial pressure from tumour usually starts as a dull, occipital pain, worse in the morning, increased with coughing or bending. Nausea, vomiting, drowsiness, and confusion develop as the intracranial pressure increases. The site of the tumour is indicated by the additional clinical signs and symptoms. Tumours seldom present with headache as a sole feature.

15 Common psychiatric disorders and psychotropic drugs

Psychiatry is the branch of medicine which is concerned with the investigation and treatment of those conditions characterized, for the main part, by abnormalities of mental state and behaviour. The separation of physical and mental aspects of illness is somewhat arbitrary in that abnormal mental states may be accompanied by physical symptoms and signs and physical illness can give rise to mental disorders.

The classification of disorders of behaviour and mental experience is limited by the lack of knowledge of the underlying cause of many conditions. Mental illness is, therefore, usually classified according to the clinical features of the illness and two main groups of disorders are recognized:

1. Personality disorders and neuroses which are the psychiatric disorders most frequently found in the general population and which shade into normal behaviour;
2. Psychoses, which are more severe forms of psychiatric disorder involving, usually, a clear change from previously normal behaviour, often accompanied by loss of contact with reality. The psychoses are divided into two main groups, the functional and the organic.

Personality disorders

The personality of an individual is a unique compound of individual personality traits. These traits are difficult to define and measure but certain traits are generally recognized, such as anxiety-proneness. A personality disorder may be identified when a particular trait is so exaggerated as to cause problems for the individual or for others. Such disorders include hysterical personality disorder, characterized by emotionally shallow and attention-seeking behaviour, and paranoid personality disorder, which applies to the abnormally suspicious and easily offended individual.

The term psychopathic personality disorder usually refers to the individual causing problems for society. The term inadequate psychopath refers to the feckless, socially disorganized individual frequently involved in petty crime. Aggressive psychopath refers to the explosive, affectionless, aggressive individual without foresight or remorse.

Management
Drug treatment is of limited value since a personality disorder is not an illness but a manifestation of personal development. Group psychotherapy may be of value in giving individuals an opportunity to experience in a controlled situation how their behaviour gives rise to problems in relation to other people and so modify their behaviour accordingly.

Neuroses
The neuroses symptoms arise from mental conflict and difficulty in adaptation to stress. Some individuals are more likely to develop neurotic symptoms than others and this vulnerability appears to be constitutionally determined. The likelihood of individuals developing neurotic symptoms is influenced by the number and nature of stressful life events that they experience and by the level of support in the environment, including quality of immediate personal relationships.

The commonest symptoms in the neuroses are anxiety and depression. Both these phenomena are entirely normal in appropriate situations but when out of proportion to the circumstances and impairing function may be considered to be neurotic symptoms. Anxiety may be described as worry, apprehension or tension and is similar to fear. Depression refers to a disorder of mood and may vary from transient 'blues' to intense and persistent misery or dejection. Four clinical types of neurotic illness are described.

Anxiety neurosis. The main complaints may be mental or physical. Physical symptoms of anxiety include palpitations, sweating, indigestion and frequency of micturition. The mental symptoms include anxiety, tension, irritability, poor concentration, difficulty getting off to sleep and intermittent depression of mood. The symptoms may develop into attacks of panic with intense anxiety, a choking sensation and a feeling of impending disaster or death.

The symptoms of anxiety may be 'free floating', that is not determined by particular circumstances, or may only arise in specific situations as in a phobic anxiety state. Phobias vary from fear of isolated items, such as spiders, to more generalized and incapacitating fears such as fear of leaving the house (agoraphobia). Dental phobia is a well recognized problem. People exhibiting dental phobia are, in general, more anxious than controls and are much more likely to have had a frightening experience in relation to dental treatment as a child reinforced by a further traumatic dental experience in their teens. They are also more likely to avoid dental treatment than controls.

Depressive neurosis. The most common complaint is depression of mood which may be accompanied by fatigue, irritability and difficulty getting off to sleep. The symptoms often fluctuate and they are frequently precipitated by social, marital and personal crises. Self-injury, especially drug overdose, is relatively common in this condition.

Hysterical neurosis. In this disorder the neurotic conflict is resolved, or at least made tolerable, by the development of a symptom which may be physical or mental. Hysterical symptoms may develop in the presence of psychotic depression or organic brain damage.

Obsessional neurosis. This is the least common of the neuroses but may cause considerable distress to the patient who is tormented by ideas or urges which he does not want and fights against. The patient often fears that he may act on his impulses or go mad.

Management

Psychotherapy and behaviour therapy are used in the management of neuroses. Psychotherapy involves establishing a relationship between patient and therapist producing modification of the patient's maladaptive behaviour through this relationship. Behaviour therapy and cognitive therapy have been developed by psychologists to assist patients in developing adaptive patterns of behaviour and extinguishing the maladaptive responses of anxiety and depression. Where social stresses play a large part in precipitating a neurotic illness involvement of a social worker may be of considerable value.

Both psychotherapy and behaviour therapy are relatively time-consuming and rapid symptomatic relief of anxiety or tension may be achieved with anxiolytic drugs such as diazepam and chlordiazepoxide. There is always a risk of drug dependence developing with these substances and the possibility of overdose must also be considered.

Functional psychoses
In the functional psychoses there is no obvious pathological lesion of the brain but investigation of possible biochemical abnormalities continues. Social and psychological factors and events such as child-birth or bereavement may act as precipitant of these disorders but the type of illness which develops appears to be constitutionally deter-mined. Two main groups of functional psychoses are described, the affective psychoses and the schizophrenias including the paranoid states.

Affective psychoses
These conditions involve abnormality of mood, either depression or, less frequently, elation. In clinical practice this psychotic type of depression is differentiated from neurotic depression on features such as later age of onset, positive family history and feelings of guilt and inadequacy. Suicide is a definite risk in a patient with psychotic depression.

The clinical features of the depressive form of the illness include depression of mood, often worse in the morning, early morning wakening with inability to go back to sleep and feelings of guilt and self-deprecation. Appetite is poor and there is often a history of weight loss. Somatic symptoms may predominate with denial of any mental symptoms and facial pain in a middle-aged woman is a well-recognized presentation of depression.

Abnormal elevation of mood, termed hypomania or mania, is an uncommon disorder and characterized by elation which may be ac-companied by irritability with over-activity and pressure of talk. The patient is insensitive and demanding, at times jocular but rapidly becoming angry when crossed.

The affective psychoses are episodic and the outlook for any individual attack is good. However, the likelihood of recurrence is high, particularly if the first attack occurs before the age of 40.

Management. An attack of psychotic depression may be treated with antidepressant drugs, or in severe cases with electroconvulsive therapy (ECT). This involves the induction of a convulsion with an electric current while the patient is under the effect of a short-acting intravenous barbiturate anaesthetic and a muscle relaxant. These forms of treatment are effective in shortening the duration of an attack of depression.

An attack of mania or hypomania may be treated with a major tranquillizer such as chlorpromazine or haloperidol and lithium carbonate is also used in the treatment of this condition.

Prophylaxis. The number of attacks of hypomania or depression may be reduced by the use of long-term treatment with lithium preparations. Good cooperation is essential as the plasma concentration of lithium must be maintained at a certain level and frequent blood sampling is necessary.

Schizophrenia and the paranoid states

Schizophrenia is a term which covers a group of serious conditions and the term implies 'splitting' with various parts of mental content functioning separately. The illness usually starts in late adolescence or early adult life and the patients may be described as previously withdrawn and isolated people. The clinical features of the illness include disorders of speech, thought, volition, perception and emotion.

The onset of the illness is gradual and emotional responses become flattened or inappropriate. Volition is reduced with loss of initiative to the point of neglect of self and work. Thought processes are impaired and speech may become incoherent. The patients may complain that their thoughts are taken away or broadcast, or that alien thoughts are put into their minds.

Hallucinations and delusions may occur. Hallucinations are sensory experiences occurring in the absence of an external stimulus and auditory hallucinations or 'voices' are the most common in schizophrenia. Delusions are false beliefs not founded in fact and not amenable to reason and are usually persecutory in nature.

The paranoid states develop insidiously, often in people who have always been over-sensitive and suspicious. The illness usually develops in middle age and the main features are delusions of a persecutory nature.

Management. Symptoms may be alleviated by a drug of the phenothiazine group such as chlorpromazine or trifluoperazine. Rehabilitation and support in the community are essential and the injectable depot preparations such as flupenthixol may be given once every two to four weeks and overcome the problem of compliance with medication following discharge from hospital.

Organic psychoses
In this group of disorders the mental symptoms and signs result from organic brain changes. The change may be acute or chronic.

The acute organic syndrome, or delirium, is seen most commonly in the very young or the old. Common precipitants are infections with raised temperature, heart failure or ingestion of cerebral depressants such as alcohol and drugs. The clinical features of delirium are clouding of consciousness with disorientation and anxiety which may develop into panic. Memory is impaired and nearby objects may be misinterpreted by the patient. The condition is reversible with treatment of the underlying cause.

The chronic organic syndrome of dementia is characterized by brain tissue change which is usually irreversible. All areas of mental function are affected with deterioration in intellect, emotional responses and personality. Onset is insidious and memory is impaired for recent events first, the patient tending to 'live in the past'. There is marked inability to learn new material or adapt to new situations. The patient becomes disorientated first in time, then in place and person. Personality change may be profound with blunting of the finer points of personality.

Aetiology of dementia
1. Degenerative disorders, e.g. senile dementia (average age of onset 75 years) and presenile dementia (onset before 65 years of age). The underlying cause of these conditions remains unknown and there is no specific treatment.
2. Cerebral arteriosclerosis often accompanied by strokes and hypertension.
3. Toxic brain damage, e.g. chronic alcoholism, lead poisoning, carbon monoxide poisoning.
4. Metabolic causes such as hypothyroidism.
5. Infections such as syphilis and herpes encephalitis.
6. Head injury.
7. Brain tumour.

Management
All cases of organic psychosis should be investigated fully and if a reversible underlying cause is found this should be treated. Where

the condition is progressive every attempt must be made to maintain functional independence in the community as long as possible but admission to an institution may become necessary.

Mental handicap

Mental handicap has been defined as a state of arrested or incomplete development of the mind including impairment of intelligence and social functioning. An IQ of less than 70 is generally accepted as consistent with mental handicap. The aetiology of mental handicap is complex but two main populations may be defined. The first includes many individuals with relatively mild mental handicap and little, if any, physical impairment. They can be considered as falling within the lower end of the normal distribution curve of intelligence within the population. The second group includes individuals with more severe mental handicap often accompanied by physical abnormalities and in this group specific aetiological factors can frequently be identified.

Genetic factors in handicap include chromosomal abnormalities as found in Down's syndrome and single gene abnormalities as in the inborn errors of metabolism such as phenylketonuria which, if detected within the first 3 months of birth, can be treated with a diet low in phenylalanine.

Infections such as rubella during pregnancy can produce mental handicap in the child and bacterial or viral meningitis or encephalitis during childhood may result in mental handicap. Trauma to the fetus during pregnancy is rare but cerebral palsy, a condition characterized by neurological abnormalities such as spasticity or athetoid movements and a variable degree of mental handicap, may be caused by trauma with intracranial haemorrhage at the time of birth.

Attitudes towards the management of mental handicap have changed from basically caring and custodial towards early detection, e.g. amniocentesis for Down's syndrome, and prevention where possible. There is more emphasis on long-term training to achieve maximum potential and optimum social functioning with support for the individual and his family in the community wherever possible.

The diagnosis of both physical illness and mental illness in the presence of severe mental handicap presents practical problems in that the individual can at times give no indication of the nature or origin of symptoms such as pain or depression. A general disturbance of behaviour may be the only indication of an underlying physical or mental illness.

Child psychiatry
The two commonest forms of psychiatric disturbance in childhood are disorders of conduct such as truanting, lying and stealing and disorders of emotion, such as fearfulness, phobias and unhappiness. Enuresis and school refusal are two common clinical problems in childhood. Psychotic illness is rare in childhood but the autistic syndrome is a form of childhood psychosis characterized by abnormality of language and withdrawal associated with mental handicap in about 70% of cases.

Childhood disorders of emotion and conduct must be assessed in relation to the child's developmental stage, as behaviour which may be entirely within the normal range at one stage of development may be grossly abnormal and require investigation and treatment at another stage of development. Factors associated with an increased risk of psychiatric disorder in childhood include low IQ, organic brain disorder, physical or mental illness in the immediate family, particularly the mother, and family discord or dysfunction. Educational, social and family factors need to be taken into account and management of chilhood psychiatric disorder includes the use of psychotherapeutic and behavioural techniques with increasing use of family therapy sessions.

Psychotropic drugs
There are now many drugs available which act on the central nervous system and are of some value in the management of psychiatric illness. The following brief classification is based on that of the World Health Organisation.

Neuroleptics (major tranquillizers)
These drugs are used most commonly in the management of psychotic illness. There are several pharmacologically distinct types of drug in this group but the most commonly used are the phenothiazines such as chlorpromazine and trifluoperazine. Haloperidol, a butyrophenone, is particularly useful in the management of mania, and thioxanthenes such as flupenthixol and clopenthixol are frequently used as depot preparations in the form of intramuscular injections for the management of chronic schizophrenia. Drug dependence is not a problem with these drugs but they may induce neurological abnormalities of an extrapyramidal type and one condition, tardive dyskenesia, may prove irreversible.

Anxiolytic sedatives (minor tranquillizers, sedatives and hypnotics). These drugs reduce anxiety and in larger doses induce sleep and usually raise the convulsive threshold. Drug dependence may develop with drugs from this group. The most widely used drugs in this group are the benzodiazepines such as chlordiazepoxide and diazepam for symptoms of anxiety and temazepam for insomnia.

Antidepressants

These drugs are used for the treatment of pathologically depressed mood, particularly of the psychotic type. There are two main types of drug in this group, the tricyclic antidepressants and more recently introduced developments of the tricyclics and the monoamine oxidase inhibitors (MAOI). The tricyclic antidepressants include imipramine and dothiepin. These drugs are commonly prescribed for depression in both general practice and hospital. Unwanted effects include dryness of the mouth, drowsiness, blurring of vision and cardiotoxicity. The newer antidepressants related to this group include mianserin and nomifensine which have fewer anticholinergic side effects and are less cardiotoxic.

The monoamine oxidase inhibitors such as phenelzine and isocarboxazid are used less commonly, usually for atypical depression with phobic features. They are not widely used in general practice because of the problems of interaction with other drugs and food substances with the need for reliable dietary control.

These three groups comprise most of the drugs in common use for psychiatric disorders. Psychostimulants such as amphetamine increase the level of alertness but are no longer in common use because of the dangers of dependence. The hallucinogens such as LSD have no place in psychiatric practice.

Drug interaction

One of the problems of the widespread use of psychotropic drugs is the interaction of these compounds with other drugs, alcohol and occasionally some foods.

Alcohol produces depression of the central nervous system and this effect is enhanced by phenothiazines, antidepressants and probably benzodiazepines. This is of practical importance in relation to drinking and driving.

The tricyclic antidepressants inhibit the effects of some hypotensive agents such as bethanidine and may enhance the pressor effects of adrenaline (epinephrine) and noradrenaline (norepinephrine).

The monoamine oxidase inhibitors (MAOI) enhance the activity of certain amines by inhibition of the enzyme normally involved in their degradation. This is of clinical importance in relation to tyramine which is found in substances such as cheese, yeast extracts and red wine. In the presence of an MAOI drug the tyramine may produce a hypertensive crisis, resulting occasionally in death. The pressor effects of adrenaline (epinephrine) and noradrenaline (norepinephrine) may be enhanced by MAOI drugs.

The monoamine oxidase inhibitors and general anaesthetic agents may interact to produce unpredictable and severe hypotension. Adverse reactions between drugs of this group and pethidine have been reported.

Local anaesthetics containing adrenaline or noradrenaline should not be used in patients using tricyclic and related antidepressants because of the enhanced risk of severe hypertension and serious cardiac arrhythmias. Prilocaine with felypressin is less likely to cause arrhythmias. The MAOI drugs enhance the pressor effects of adrenaline and noradrenaline but do not potentiate their arrhythmic effect.

16 Common infectious diseases

Whooping cough (pertussis)

Organism. *Bordetella pertussis*

Spread. Droplet infection

Incubation period. 7–14 days

Clinical features. Children under five years are most susceptible. The disease is particularly severe in children under six months of age. After the incubation period the child develops catarrh and a mild cough. By the second week of the illness the catarrh has usually cleared but the cough has become worse and is now paroxysmal and is followed by the characteristic whooping sound. Thick tenacious mucus is usually expectorated or vomited up at the end of a spasm of coughing. The whooping stage may last for several weeks, gradual recovery then takes place.

Complications. These include bronchopneumonia, lung collapse (atelectasis), and very occasionally bronchiectasis. Nose bleeds and haemoptysis may occur during a spasm and ulceration of the frenulum of the tongue may follow trauma by the lower teeth.

Treatment. Bordetella pertussis in vitro is sensitive to a number of antibiotics. In the established disease, however, antibiotic therapy has proved very disappointing.

Prophylaxis. See schedule of immunization (p.108). It is worth noting that mild attacks of whooping cough may still occur in immunized children.

Measles (morbilli)

Organism.   Measles virus

Spread.   Droplet infection

Incubation period.   10–11 days

Clinical features. The illness starts with severe catarrhal symptoms. On the second day Koplik's spots appear on the buccal and lower mucosa and around the openings of the parotid ducts. These spots are like grains of salt, surrounded by a small area of inflammation. The Koplik's spots disappear in three to four days. The skin rash, which is a dark red maculopapular eruption, appears on the fourth day of illness and spreads rapidly to cover the whole body. The rash fades over the course of about a week.

Complications. These are usually due to secondary bacterial infection and include bronchopneumonia, otitis media and gastroenteritis. Encephalitis is a rare but serious complication.

Treatment. Antibiotics should be reserved for secondary bacterial infection.

Prophylaxis. Active immunization is with live attenuated measles vaccine. Pooled human gamma globulin is sometimes used to give short-term protection to children exposed to measles infection.

German measles (rubella)

Organism.   Rubella virus

Spread.   Droplet infection

Incubation period.   18–19 days

Clinical features. Rubella is a mild illness with very few complications. A pink maculopapular rash appears on the second day of illness. The rash covers the whole body. It fades in a few days. Early in the illness there is mild inflammation of the throat and palate, and the posterior cervical lymph nodes are usually enlarged and tender. Recovery is rapid in children. Adults may have a slightly more prolonged illness.

Treatment. None is required.

Prevention. Girls aged 11–13 yrs should receive rubella vaccine. Women found to have no antibodies to rubella during pregnancy should be given the vaccine immediately after delivery to ensure protection during subsequent pregnancies. Vaccine must not be given during pregnancy.

Notes. A rash very similar to rubella may be present in other viral illnesses, e.g. glandular fever, echovirus infection and human parvovirus infection. If rubella develops in a patient who is in the first four months of pregnancy the fetus may die and be aborted or if it survives it may be born with congenital abnormalities caused by rubella virus.

Mumps

Organism. Mumps virus

Spread. Droplet infection—contact with infected saliva

Incubation period. 18–21 days

Clinical features. Mumps virus usually causes inflammation of the salivary glands—the parotid gland being most often affected. Other glands may however be involved; these include the pancreas, the sex glands (adults only) and the thyroid gland. The virus may also attack the meninges and the brain giving rise to meningitis and/or encephalitis. In children the disease is usually more severe particularly if the sex glands are involved. Orchitis in the male may be unilateral or bilateral. Sterility may follow mumps orchitis but fortunately this rarely happens.

Treatment. This is symptomatic with particular attention being paid to mouth hygiene.

Orchitis may subside more rapidly if the patient is given a short course of steroid therapy.

Prophylaxis. A live attenuated mumps virus vaccine is available now but it is not given routinely to children in Britain. It can be used to protect males who have not had mumps by the time they reach puberty.

Chickenpox (varicella)

Organism. Varicella virus

Spread. Droplet infection and contact with spots in the early stages of the disease

Incubation period. 14–15 days

Clinical features. Chickenpox is a mild illness especially in children. Vesicles first appear in the mouth, especially on the palate where they rupture rapidly to form shallow painful oval ulcers. The rash on the skin consists of macules which rapidly change to papules and then to oval-shaped vesicles. Pustules form within 48 hours. These dry up and scab over. The scabs separate without leaving scars unless the spots have been made deeper by scratching. Following an attack of chickenpox some virus particles may remain latent in the body. These may become active again after many years and give rise to herpes zoster (shingles).

Complications. Secondary sepsis of the chickenpox lesions. Encephalitis is a very rare but serious complication of chickenpox.

Treatment. No treatment is required, but if possible children should be prevented from scratching the spots.

Acute infectious diarrhoea
Diarrhoeal illness is still a frequent cause of morbidity and occasionally of mortality in Britain. Infecting agents include the Shigella group of organisms which cause dysentery, Campylobacter species and viruses such as rotavirus which is the commonest cause of diarrhoea in infants and young children. Food infection with Salmonella organisms, *Staphylococcus aureus* or *Clostridium welchii* may cause large or small outbreaks of sickness and diarrhoea. Typhoid and paratyphoid (the enteric fevers) are now no longer endemic in Britain. These diseases may still, however, be imported by travellers from overseas and it is still most important that people travelling from this country to areas where the enteric fevers are endemic should be adequately protected by immunization with monovalent typhoid vaccine.

Management of acute diarrhoeal illness
Most important is the maintenance of hydration with oral or intravenous fluids. Electrolyte imbalance must be corrected. In most

cases of infectious diarrhoea, antibiotics are not required and may even do harm. Exceptions are Campylobacter infections which respond well to erythromycin and the enteric fevers which require treatment with chloramphenicol or cotrimoxazole.

Influenza

Organism. Influenza virus type A or B

Spread. Droplet infection

Incubation period. 12–48 hours

Clinical features. Influenza tends to occur in epidemics and is very highly infectious. The virus attacks the mucous membranes of the upper respiratory tract. Many of the complications of influenza are due to super-infection with bacteria such as *Haemophilus influenzae*, *Streptococcus pneumoniae* and *Staphylococcus aureus*. The patient presents with fever, malaise, sore throat, headache, cough and myalgia. The fauces and pharynx are inflamed but there is usually no exudate on the tonsils. The illness is self-limiting and lasts 4–5 days. In elderly and debilitated patients influenza and its complications may cause fatal illness. Death is often due to associated bacterial pneumonia.

Treatment. There is no specific treatment for ordinary influenza. Antibiotic therapy should be reserved for control of secondary bacterial infection.

Prophylaxis. Immunization with influenza vaccine offers some protection but because the virus is constantly producing new antigenic variants, repeated vaccination is required preferably using strains of the virus expected to cause epidemics. The anti-viral agent amantadine has been used prophylactically with some success to protect elderly or debilitated patients exposed to influenza A virus.

Tuberculosis *See also* p.58.

Organism. Mycobacterium tuberculosis.

Clinical features. The incidence of tuberculosis has fallen markedly in Britain in recent years as a result of improved social conditions,

more effective anti-tuberculous therapy, mass miniature radiography and vigorous contact tracing. New cases are, however, still being identified, particularly in the older age group. Especially at risk of developing tuberculosis are debilitated patients, diabetics, patients on steroid therapy and those patients, who through disease or as a result of drug therapy, are immuno-suppressed. The incidence is also high in some immigrant populations because of low 'herd' immunity in the community. Tuberculosis may involve the lungs in the following ways:
1. *Asymptomatic* self-limiting primary infection.
2. *Cavitating chronic infection,* typically involving the upper lobes, giving a chronic cough, often with fever and haemoptysis and weight loss.
3. *Pleural effusion.*
4. *Bronchial obstruction* due to external pressure from enlarged lymph nodes or to blockage from within by granulation tissue.
5. *Bronchiectasis.*
6. *Tuberculous bronchopneumonia.* Spread of the organisms from the lung via the blood stream to involve other organs may occur, e.g. renal tuberculosis, tuberculosis of bones and joints, and tuberculous meningitis. Miliary tuberculosis is the result of widespread blood dissemination of tubercle bacilli throughout the lungs and other organs.

Diagnosis is confirmed by identification of the organism either by direct microscopy or by culture from sputum in pulmonary TB, or from urine, CSF, stool, or joint fluid in non-pulmonary forms of tuberculosis.

Note. The Mantoux test becomes positive following the primary infection.

Treatment. Antituberculous drugs should always be used in combination to avoid the emergence of drug resistance. The drugs most often used include isoniazid, rifampicin, ethambutol and streptomycin. For choice of drug combination and principles of therapy *see* p.60. Surgical treatment is now rarely required for pulmonary tuberculosis.

Glandular fever (infectious mononucleosis).
See p.288.

17 The elderly

Demography

In the present century there has been a dramatic rise in the proportion of old people in the UK (Table 5). Between 1971 and the end of this century the proportion aged between 65 and 74 will level out, but that for people of 75 and over will continue to rise.

This change in the age structure has important implications for the organization of health care. An example is that the proportion of people having problems with activities of daily living is 2% for those aged less than 65, rising to 10% for those aged 65 to 74, and 20% for those aged 75 and over.

Table 5. Percentage of total population aged over 65 years in Great Britain between 1901 and 2001.

Age in years	1901	1931	1971	2001
65 – 74	3.2	5.4	8.3	8.0
75 +	1.6	2.1	4.0	6.2
Total	4.8	7.5	12.3	14.2

Ageing and physiological function

Muscles

Ageing is associated with a progressive decline in muscle mass and muscle power. This is partly the result of denervations following neuronal death. (Nerve cells unlike epithelial cells are unable to divide themselves, so that death of an individual neurone results in an irreversible reduction in the total number of neurones.) An additional factor is the decline in activity associated with ageing so that, even in old age, some of the reduction in muscle power can be corrected by an appropriate programme of physical exercise.

Sensation
There also is a decline in touch, pain, vibration and position sense. The decline in position sense means that old people rely increasingly on vision to maintain balance and are thus in difficulty if their eyesight is poor or their surroundings are poorly lit. A decline in deep pain sensation means that disorders involving viscera, e.g. myocardial infarction, cholelithiasis, may present in an atypical or less dramatic fashion.

Hearing
Ageing results in degeneration of the cochlea with specific changes in hearing. These are as follows:
1. There is selective impairment of high frequency receptors, so that consonants are less easily heard than vowels. Compensate for this by articulating clearly!
2. There is selective damage of low amplitude as opposed to loud amplitude receptors. Loud sounds are therefore uncomfortable and distorted. Speak up but don't shout!
3. Processing of sound information is slowed. Speak slowly!
4. The ability to 'focus' on sound is lost, particularly if a hearing aid is used. Avoid conversations in a noisy environment!
5. Visual clues become important. Talk to the patient facing him and in a good light.

Taste and smell
There is a decline in both taste and smell sensation. The problem is accentuated if the patient is a heavy smoker or drinker, has oral infections, is on drugs interfering with salivation, or has poor oral hygiene.

Vision
There are a variety of visual changes:
1. *Loss of lens elasticity.* This occurs in early middle age and causes long sightedness so that the subject requires reading glasses.
2. *Lens opacity.* This occurs in old age and can be corrected by removal of the lens.
3. Common eye diseases in old age include *glaucoma* (high intraocular pressure) and *macular degeneration* (destruction of the central part

of the retina). These respond to treatment if identified before irreversible retinal damage has occurred.

Autonomic nervous system

Changes in the function of the autonomic nervous system in old age produce several important disorders:

1. *Postural hypotension.* Degeneration of the sympathetic nervous system means that when an elderly person stands up the blood vessels in his legs do not constrict and his heart rate does not increase. Blood pools in his legs resulting in a fall in cerebral perfusion, and a feeling of faintness or dizziness.
2. *Hypothermia.* Inadequate constriction of subcutaneous vessels means that an elderly patient continues to radiate heat during cold weather. The process is accentuated by a wide range of drugs and disease.
3. *Irritable bladder.* Loss of inhibitory fibres from the cerebral cortex to the bladder produces an organ which is small, has a high internal pressure and empties frequently. This may give rise to the symptoms of urinary frequency, nocturia and incontinence. Other causes of these include a lax urethral sphincter, and an enlarged prostate.

Cardiorespiratory reserve

A variety of histological changes in heart muscle such as lipofuscin deposition, fibrosis and amyloidosis mean that the stroke volume and maximum heart rate are reduced. Degeneration of inter-alveolar connective tissue means that lung elasticity is reduced and ventilatory capacity compromised.

These changes cause no problems under *baseline* conditions, but doing physical exercise reduces the rate at which oxygen can be delivered to vital tissues (maximum oxygen consumption).

Though an age-related decline in maximum oxygen consumption is inevitable, the rate at which this occurs can be reduced by taking regular exercise. It is accelerated by cigarette smoking.

Excretion and metabolism

1. Despite a progressive decline in renal function, old people have sufficient reserve capacity to maintain homeostasis under baseline conditions. They respond poorly to stress. Diarrhoea, diuretic treatment, or an inadequate intake of fluid all may lead to severe

dehydration. Many drugs are eliminated by the kidney so that if standard doses are given to old people, toxic blood levels may result.
2. Some forms of hepatic enzyme activity are reduced. This again may cause toxicity if drugs metabolized by the liver are given in too large a dose.

Illness in old age
Ageing has a relatively trivial effect on physical capacity in old age compared with the striking effect which diseases common in old age have upon this.

Multiple pathology
Many old people suffer from more than a dozen different disorders at once. This complicates the business of fitting signs and symptoms together to produce diagnoses. Multiple disorders lead to multiple investigations. Only investigate if a positive or negative result will alter patient management. Multiple pathology leads to polypharmacy. There is a geometrical rise in the incidence of drug side effects with the number of drugs used. (A patient on eight drugs is 64 times more likely to have side effects than a patient on one drug.) Only use a drug if the benefits outweigh the risk of side effects.

Disability
Diseases in old people are much more likely to interfere with mobility and self-care capacity than those in a younger group. The following are examples:

Stroke. This characteristically produces weakness down the one side but is also associated with a wide range of other symptoms including dysphasia, hemianopia, sensory disturbances, impaired balance and urinary dysfunction. Rehabilitation requires the coordinated efforts of the doctor, nurse, physiotherapist, occupational therapist and speech therapist. The social worker is then involved in resolving the social and psychological problems posed by any residual incapacity.

An issue of particular interest to dentists is that stroke patients experience problems with dentures and these may have to be modified. There may be swallowing difficulties and exercises organized by a speech therapist are useful here. Finally, drooling from the paralysed side of the mouth is often an embarrassing problem. *See also* p.172.

Parkinsonism. This is characterized by poverty of movement, rigidity and a tremor. Patients have a mask-like face, a stooped posture, and a shuffling gait in which they always seem to be chasing their centre of gravity.

Orofacial problems include a soft indistinct voice, difficulty in swallowing, and dribbling as a result of hypersalivation.

The condition shows a gratifying response to replacement therapy using l-dopa. Overdosage of this can produce peculiar writhing movements of the tongue and lips (orofacial dyskinesia). *See also* p.175.

Osteoarthritis. This condition, characterized by degeneration of cartilage and elimination of bone underlying joint surfaces, is almost universal in the hips and knees. Surprisingly, there is little correlation between the degree of pain or disability caused by the disorder and the severity of radiological changes. If, because of pain and stiffness, patients are allowed to become immobile it is often difficult to restore function. It is important, therefore, to refer patients with early symptoms of osteoarthritis to a geriatric day hospital so that with an appropriate analgesic regime and course of physiotherapy permanent incapacity may be prevented.

Surgical joint replacement is useful in more severe cases. Limiting factors are severe mental or physical incapacity, poor quality of surrounding bone, and long orthopaedic waiting lists. *See also* p.156.

Osteoporosis. Bone rarefaction is almost universal in old age and is particularly severe in women. It may cause collapse of a vertebral body resulting in pain and kyphotic deformity. The process also involves the proximal femur and fractures of this place a heavy load on orthopaedic departments. Not only do they form a major part of the surgical workload, but the physical and mental disorders often accompanying the fractures often mean that rehabilitation and discharge are extremely difficult requiring close co-ordination with the geriatric service. *See also* p.150.

Presentation of disease

Heart disease. A large number of old people suffer from heart disease. Hypertension, angina on exertion, congestive cardiac failure and valvular disorders are all common problems. Both the disorders themselves and drugs used in their treatment cause a great deal of morbidity, so that dentists should always check on whether an old person has heart disease and whether he is on digoxin, a diuretic or a β-adrenoceptor blocker.

Subacute bacterial endocarditis, a particular complication of valvular heart disease, is especially common in old age. Appropriate antibiotic cover before dental treatment is therefore indicated. Once the condition becomes established, the symptoms and signs, though severe, are often vague and atypical and go unrecognized (p.36).

Chest infections are particularly dangerous in old age. Impaired immunological function means that a bronchopneumonia spreads rapidly in a patient further compromised by a reduced cardiorespiratory reserve. A further problem is that an increased pain threshold and immunological incompetence mean that the condition often presents in an uncharacteristic way. Rather than complaining of breathlessness and showing signs of a consolidation, the patient may be muddled and feel tired. Other infections involving the gallbladder, appendix or urinary tract may also present in the same undramatic way. Yet another condition often presenting atypically is myocardial infarction, where central chest pain may be absent.

Hypothyroidism. Features of this condition include mental slowing, coarse features, hair loss, a hoarse voice, intolerance of cold, a slow pulse and constipation. Ageing produces a similar pattern of abnormalities so that, in old people, hypothyroidism is often missed. A high level of suspicion is required to identify and treat this potentially reversible condition. *See also* p.139.

Diabetes mellitus is extremely common in old age but often presents insidiously so that it is easily missed. The easiest way of picking it up is to check the blood glucose concentration in a random sample of blood. The condition is responsible for a wide range of chronic problems (Table 6). Acute manifestations such as ketosis, hyperosmolar coma and lactic acidosis do occur but are less common. *See* also p.129.

Mental impairment
Throughout adult life there is a progressive decline in the number of brain cells. Like most other cells, however, there is a considerable

excess of numbers over requirements even in old age. This means that ageing has relatively little effect on mental function. Many of the psychological differences between young and old people are a cohort effect; that is, old people come from a different cultural background, had different educational standards, and were exposed to different health risks and nutritional standards.

A minority of old people suffer from diseases causing diffuse cerebral destruction associated with mental impairment. The proportions of old people with severe mental impairment between 65 and 74, 75 and 84, and 85 and over are 2%, 10% and 25% respectively.

The most common cause of mental impairment in old age is Alzheimer's disease, a condition characterized in the cortex by large plaques of degenerative material (senile plaques) and neurones containing tangles of microtubules (neurofibrillary tangles). Mental impairment may also be the result of multiple small cerebral infarcts. Lastly, there is a small but important group of patients with mental impairment due to reversible conditions such as hypothyroidism, hypoglycaemia or normal pressure hydrocephalus. *See also* pp.139 & 192.

Table 6 Complications of diabetes mellitus in old age.

Eyes	cataract
	retinopathy
Mouth	candidosis
Lungs	tuberculosis
	bronchopneumonia
Heart	myocardial ischaemia
Brain	cerebrovascular disease
Kidneys	nephrotic syndrome
	pyelonephritis
	cystitis
Vagina	candidosis
Legs	peripheral vascular disease
	peripheral neuropathy (trophic ulcer)
Skin	candidosis

Dental problems
It is a common misconception that because many old people have no teeth, old people have little need of a dentist. Table 7 indicates that old people in fact have a wide range of dental problems.

Unfortunately, because of multiple pathology and disability, many old people in need of dental care are unable to get to a surgery. New strategies are required to cope with what will be a steadily increasing problem.

Table 7.   Dental status of old people living at home.

Proportion of subjects who are edentulous	74%
Proportion of edentulous subjects with dentures	98%
Proportion of edentulous subjects with satisfactory dentures	10%
Proportion of subjects with oral lesions	60%
Proportion of dentulous with caries	40%
Proportion of dentulous with gingivitis	60%

18 Renal and urinary disorders and organ transplantation

The kidneys and the urine-conduction system comprise a functional unit which is concerned with the preservation of the normal composition and volume of the extracellular fluid by regulating the excretion of water and water-soluble solids. Disease of this system (the ureters, bladder, prostate [in the male] and the urethra) can either manifest locally or by affecting kidney function. The diseases of the urinary passages are protean. The common disorders of the system are infection, neoplasm or the result of mechanical obstruction to urine flow. Obstruction almost always leads to infection. Table 8 lists the commonest conditions. Biochemistry, contrast radiology and endoscopy are the methods of investigation used to elicit the precise diagnosis.

Prolonged obstruction of urine flow can, by 'back pressure', eventually impair renal function, the process being termed *obstructive uropathy*. Since obstruction is often compounded by infection the involvement of the renal parenchyma by inflammatory infiltration is often present (*pyelonephritis*).

Disorders of the kidneys
These comprise almost all the known pathological processes—congenital defects (*agenesis, hypoplasia*), *acute and chronic infection* (*E. coli, S. aureus, M. tuberculosis*), *hypertensive injury (nephropathy)*, *diabetic microangiopathy*, *infarction* by embolism and benign and malignant neoplasms (*renal adenoma* and *carcinoma*). In addition, the glomeruli, which are unique ultra-filters for blood plasma, are prone to a spectrum of inflammatory processes which result from the impaction within them of antibodies, immune complexes and inflammatory products arising from disease processes outwith the kidney. These materials which are derived from the blood stream and ultimately from the immune system are deposited in the capillary walls of the glomeruli. These various inflammatory glomerular

211

illnesses are not associated with the presence of micro-organisms within the glomeruli, although antigens from bacteria and viruses may play a part in their development. These illnesses are termed *glomerulonephritis*.

Damage to the kidney may present with haematuria, proteinuria, a renal mass, pain in the loin or flank, or simply and most commonly with the syndrome of chronic (azotaemic) renal failure.

Table 8   Disorders of the urinary passages.

	Pathology	Mechanism	Clinical expression
Pelvis of ureter	Stone formation (nephrolithiasis)	Deposition of urinary salts (calcium oxalate and phosphate)	Loin pain, predisposition to infection
Ureter	Calculus	Obstruction	Ureteric colic
	Stricture fibrous or neoplastic	Obstruction	Ureteric colic
Bladder	Acute cystitis	*E. coli* infections	Dysuria and increased frequency of micturition
	Chronic cystitis	*E. coli; M.* tuberculosis	Dysuria and increased frequency of micturition
	Papilloma	Benign neoplasia	Painless haematuria
	Incontinence and/or retention of urine	Various, e.g. overflow with chronic bladder distension or denervation	Poor urine stream, soiling of urine
Prostate	Benign hyperplasia Carcinoma	Urethral obstruction	Retention of urine
Urethra	Urethritis	*N. gonococcus,* non-specific infections	Purulent discharge from urinary meatus or dysuria

Clinical syndromes, renal insufficiency (azotaemia) and uraemia
The impairment of renal function results in chemical disorganization of the extracellular fluid and, indirectly, affects cell function throughout the body. Of the many components involved, retained urea, creatinine and non-volatile acids are most readily measured in the serum. Alterations in the urine also occur such as changes in its production rate (volume) or protein or cell content. Increases in the serum urea and creatinine concentrations (normal ranges 3–6 mmol/l and 70–120 μmol/l respectively) inversely reflect reduction

in glomerular filtration and commonly loss of functional renal tissue. Early on this may not be evident clinically. There are six main patterns of renal insufficiency clinically recognizable (Table 9). The terms *acute* and *chronic* refer to the tempo of the disease process and the accompanying clinical illness. Those termed acute operate in a time scale of days or weeks. The more frequent chronic ones advance over many months or years, even decades, usually being preceded by a long asymptomatic phase. The commonest form of renal insufficiency is *chronic (azotaemic) renal failure (CARF)* which is usually recognized belatedly after an insidious beginning with vague ill-health. Brief descriptions of the six main syndromes are as follows:

Table 9 Clinical varieties or renal impairment.

	Asymptomatic	Symptomatic
Acute		Oliguric/anuric renal failure (renal tubular necrosis)
		Acute nephritic syndrome (acute glomerulonephritis)
Chronic	Mild proteinuria and/or microhaematuria	Nephrotic syndrome (gross proteinuria with oedema)
	Minimal azotaemia Normochromic, normocytic anaemia	Chronic (azotaemic) renal failure ↓
	Mild – moderate hypertension	End-stage renal failure ↓ Uraemia

Oliguric/anuric renal failure

This acute illness develops in the wake of prolonged severe circulatory impairment (e.g. traumatic shock or exposure to nephro-toxins such as paraquat or gentamicin). The lesion consists of patchy necrosis of the renal tubular epithelium with preserved glomeruli giving it the alternative name of *renal tubular necrosis*. Urine output is characteristically reduced to less than 400 ml/24 hours for one to two weeks. This is followed by gradual recovery of full renal function provided that the patient survives the acute illness. Death may occur early from hyperkalaemia. Dialysis therapy can often tide the patient over the acute phase of illness until the tubular injury and function recovers. This illness always necessitates hospital admission and management.

Acute nephritic syndrome
This is an acute form of glomerulonephritis. Immune complexes, formed as a result of antecedent bacterial or viral infection, but especially streptococcal tonsillitis, deposit in glomerular capillary walls and cause a local inflammatory reaction. Micro-organisms are not present in the glomeruli, but antigens combined with antibodies to these antigens deposit as immune complexes. This results in oedema (commonly facial), diastolic arterial hypertension and oliguria with smokey-brown haematuria. The process is self-limiting after two or three weeks, usually with complete recovery of renal function and no aftermath.

Nephrotic syndrome
Increased permeability of the glomerulus to serum proteins, particularly albumin, results in proteinuria. In small amounts the proteinuria is detectable only on chemical analysis of the urine. If rather more than 5 g of protein are lost in the urine daily, the patient develops hypoalbuminaemia and then ankle swelling. The dependent symmetrical oedema can become gross. Some of these patients are even oedematous up to waist level. Each patient becomes grossly protein-depleted and is prone to infection as a result of hypogammaglobulinaemia. There are many causes of the nephrotic syndrome. In children, the commonest is *lipoid nephrosis* (*minimal change nephropathy*) and this is responsive to corticosteroid therapy, although relapses are common. Lipoid nephrosis is not followed by end-stage renal failure. In adults glomerulonephritis is the common underlying cause of the nephrotic syndrome and the course is often prolonged. In many adults the nephrotic syndrome is followed by the development of hypertension and chronic (azotaemic) renal failure. The time course may extend over many months or one or two years.

Chronic (azotaemic) renal failure
This common illness begins insidiously as vague ill-health. The early half of the illness is featureless except for possible non-renal expression of the causative process, e.g. headaches in *analgesic nephropathy* or skin rash and arthropathy in *lupus erythematosus*. The clinical expression of the renal involvement is indirect and often misleading. Commonly alimentary upsets (nausea, recurrent vomiting, and sometimes diarrhoea) are usually associated with hypertension and a normochromic anaemia. The renal features are inconspicuous and may consist only of the need to pass urine overnight (*nocturia*),

reflecting an increased urine volume (*polyuria*), with resultant accompanying thirst (*polydipsia*). Physical features are few. A generalized muddy-yellow pigmentation of the skin and a generalized itch are usual in the later stages. Clinical suspicion of the disorder is confirmed by finding increased serum creatinine and urea levels (*azotaemia*). The recognition of CARF is but a part-diagnosis. It is essential that the underlying cause of the renal impairment be discovered. The three commonest causes are chronic glomerulonephritis, chronic pyelonephritis and obstructive prostatic disease.

End-stage renal failure
Progressive chronic (azotaemic) renal failure passes into end-stage renal failure. This is a profound illness affecting even bone and nerve function, as well as haemopoietic tissue, the immune response and haemostasis. Finally uraemia supervenes.

Uraemia
This is the name given to the terminal phase of renal failure. It is characterized by a bed-bound wasting state with dull consciousness, muscle twitching, recurrent vomiting and deep, hissing (*acidotic*) respiration. In this state there is a foul uriniferous odour on the breath accompanying stomatitis. The patient is obviously gravely ill and develops an aseptic inflammation of the pericardium which signals that death is likely to occur within a matter of days or weeks.

Treatment
In general, there are two aspects to the treatment of renal disorders. The first is *curative* directed at the cause. The second is *conservative* or *symptomatic*, aimed at retarding or reversing the consequences of the renal insufficiency. Curative treatment is comparatively common in the diseases of the renal parenchyma. Antibiotics fall within this category, as does antihypertensive therapy, steroids for minimal change nephropathy and surgical removal of obstruction in the urinary tract strictures, ureteric stones and the like. Symptomatic treatment is used for renal disorders which have no recognized cure such as glomerulonephritis.

In its early stages (i.e. when serum urea is less than 25 mmol/l) chronic azotaemic renal failure needs no symptomatic treatment. When more advanced, the main line of therapy lies in dietary manipulation. Reduced protein intake eliminates azotaemic vomiting and restores appetite so long as sufficient fat and carbohydrate food can be ingested to obviate any emerging calorie deficit. When the serum urea is greater than 30 mmol/l the daily protein intake may be restricted to 40 g of first-class sources daily. Calorie supplements are then essential. When successful, the gastrointestinal symptoms disappear but the patient remains anaemic and the glomerular filtration rate (GFR) is unaffected. Such patients are readily upset by intercurrent stress, e.g. anaesthetic-induced vomiting, gastroenteritis, and some drugs, e.g. tetracycline. Medication has relatively little place in the treatment of chronic (azotaemic) renal failure but the renal failure has a major influence upon drug treatment of concomitant other medical or surgical conditions in the same patient. It is also noteworthy that patients over 60 years of age have an age-related deterioration in GFR which affects dosage with urine-excreted drugs such as digoxin, the cephalosporins, and the aminoglycosides such as gentamicin or netilmicin.

End-stage renal failure: dialysis and transplantation
Permanent (irreversible) renal failure can be counteracted by haemodialysis treatment and ultimately by *renal transplantation*. Maintenance dialysis involves regular treatment sessions with the patient connected to an artificial kidney for two or three 5-hour periods every week or recurrent infusions of sterile fluid by the patient into the peritoneum (*continuous ambulatory peritoneal dialysis—CAPD*). Both forms of treatment must be continued indefinitely or until successful kidney transplant eventuates. The two dialysis modalities restore a measure of health and permit a return to normal diet. Neither form of substitution therapy provides robust health as these patients generally remain significantly anaemic.

Renal transplantation is generally favoured over dialysis for the long-term but not every patient can hope to receive a transplant kidney because of tissue-matching problems and especially because of the shortage of donation of suitable cadaver kidneys. All patients for kidney transplants have a multi-drug regimen including steroids (prednisolone) and immunosuppression (azathioprine or cyclosporin). These patients in particular are susceptible to opportunistic infections such as cytomegalovirus, wart virus, *pneumocystis carinii* and drug toxicity effects.

Dental practice and renal/urinary disorders
From the dental view-point the chronic renal failure patients may look reasonably normal but are nearly always severely anaemic and

hypertensive or occasionally hypotensive. Local conservative dental treatment is not contra-indicated except in late renal failure, that is near-uraemia.

Caution is required when dealing with patients on dialysis and those with kidney transplants. Those on haemodialysis are heparinized with each treatment session and dental treatment should be coordinated with the dialysis to avoid the period of maximum effect of the heparin. CAPD does not involve systemic heparinization and if the patient feels well, local treatment in the mouth including extractions can proceed normally. It is advisable, however, to check with the renal unit concerned to obtain the information upon the recent haemoglobin level and other features which may be peculiar to the individual patient.

In the past and, much less commonly, now, patients on dialysis therapy or who have been on dialysis therapy, have been prone to contract hepatitis B and to become carriers of that virus. This largely resulted from the practice of multiple transfusions to try and overcome anaemia. A decade ago the blood used for these transfusions was not screened for hepatitis B and, as a result, some of the patients contracted the infection. Certain outbreaks of hepatitis in dialysis units received national attention and in some cases the staff were affected. The UK dialysis units are largely free of this problem at present because of a policy of minimal blood transfusions complemented by the careful screening of the patients and any blood used for hepatitis B. Despite this improved position, it is generally prudent to avoid direct contact with the dialysis patient's blood when undertaking procedures in the mouth. When the patient's serum is positive for HBsAg (Australia antigen) it is the policy in some areas to refer patients on dialysis to dental hospitals for other than the simplest procedures. When the patient is is HBs Ag positive it is clearly prudent for the dentist to wear gloves and goggles when dental treatment is being administered.

Organ transplantation

One of the most recent developments in surgery is the transplanting of organs from one person to another. Currently this is at a stage where cornea and kidney transplantation is established and accepted, liver and heart transplantations are looking promising and pancreas and lung transplantations are being tried. These advances have come about not only because of the development of surgical techniques but because of the parallel development of tissue-typing and methods of controlled immunosuppression.

Initially organs for transplantation were obtained from deceased persons, after circulatory arrest, or from living close relatives. The former method was associated with a high incidence of transplantation of irreversibly damaged organs, and the second with high emotional costs.

The more recent development of a method of diagnosing death of the brain before circulatory arrest has facilitated donation of organs. The viability of these organs is considerably greater than those taken after an interval of cardiac arrest, because the warm ischaemic time is substantially reduced and autolysis diminished. Many members of the public now carry on their persons a card indicating their consent to their organs being taken for transplantation at their death. Untimely death such as might ensue from an accident or injury can often mean that organs which are likely to be successfully transplanted are available. Such patients may be maintained on a life support system until it is ascertained, using the appropriate tests carried out by two independent clinicians on two separate occasions, that there is no function of the brain stem. Certain legal procedures must be completed, especially where injury was involved, but society, coming to recognise the value of transplantation, is accepting the need to facilitate these and usually the responsible coroner or procurator fiscal will do all in his power to enable donated organs to be transplanted.

The diagnostic tests for confirmation of brain death are the absence of all brain-stem reflexes, as follows:
1. The pupils are fixed in diameter and do not respond to sharp changes in the intensity of incidental light,
2. There is no corneal reflex,
3. The vestibulo-ocular reflexes are absent,
4. There is no gag reflex response to bronchial stimulation by a suction catheter passed down the trachea,
5. No respiratory movements occur when the patient is disconnected from the mechanical ventilator for long enough to ensure that the arterial carbon dioxide tension rises above the threshold for stimulation of respiration.

The dentist needs to remember the possibilty that patients may have undergone a transplant and be on some form of immunosuppression therapy that could predispose to infection or delay wound healing.

19 Principles of clinical pharmacology

For centuries, medical therapeutic practice consisted of using crude substances from animal, plant or mineral sources in a traditional and empirical way. These preparations contained variable amounts of pharmacologically active agents. More recently, not only have an increasing number of drugs become available, but these are usually now chemically synthesized and the drug therapy is now evaluated more scientifically, aided by an increased understanding of the pathophysiology of disease processes.

Drug action

Drugs may act in a number of different ways. Some may act on specific receptors, macromolecular structures which are linked to effector mechanisms. This drug–receptor interaction may result in stimulation or blockade of the receptor. Drugs which stimulate receptors are called *agonists*, e.g. the sympathomimetic amines isoprenaline and adrenaline; drugs which block receptors are *antagonists*, and this antagonism may be either reversible or *competitive*, or non-reversible or *non-competitive*. Competitive antagonism blocks the effect of an agonist at a receptor site and can be overcome by increasing the amount of agonist, e.g. the effects of the β-adrenoceptor blocking drug, propranolol, can be counteracted by the β-adrenoceptor agonist, isoprenaline. Non-competitive antagonism cannot be overcome by increasing the appropriate agonist concentration, and recovery depends on the synthesis of new receptors, e.g. phenoxybenzamine irreversibly blocks α-adrenoceptors.

Drugs may act by interacting with enzymes, enhancing or inhibiting activity. Again the interaction may be competitive (or reversible), e.g. cimetidine competitively inhibits H_2-histamine receptors: it may also be *non-competitive* and irreversible, e.g. the inhibition of prostaglandin synthetase by aspirin.

Drugs may also influence ionic movements and hence transmembrane potentials across cell walls: common examples of drugs that work in this way are anti-arrhythmic agents. Some drugs damage or kill micro-organisms or malignant cells by a variety of mechanisms, including effects on specific receptors or enzymes, or damage to DNA: antibiotics and anti-cancer drugs may work like this.

Drug administration
The way in which a drug is administered is determined by a number of factors. These include speed of onset needed, site of action required, absorption of drug from the gastrointestinal tract and expertise available. Oral administration is simple, safe, cheap and most pleasant for the patient. However, some drugs can be applied directly to their site of action, e.g. topical application of fungicides to infected skin and bronchodilator inhalation in asthmatics. Intravenous (i.v.) administration results in rapid attainment of high drug levels in blood and is the route of choice for some drugs in seriously ill patients. Drugs may also be given intramuscularly (i.m.), intra-arterially (i.a.), subcutaneously (s.c.), sublingually (s.l.), and rectally (p.r.).

Drug absorption
The most important mechanism for drug absorption at the cellular level is passive diffusion. This is determined by the concentration gradient and by the ability of the drug to cross a cell membrane. Fat-soluble, un-ionized drugs are well-absorbed; water-soluble, ionized substances pass through cell membranes less readily.

Some drugs are well absorbed from the gut lumen but are then extensively metabolized either in the gut wall or on their 'first-pass' through the liver. Such drugs may have to be given by another mechanism, e.g. lignocaine is given parenterally and glyceryl trinitrate is used sublingually; others, particularly those used for pain relief, like pentazocine and morphine, require to be given in a larger dose when used orally than when used intravenously.

Drug distribution
Once a drug has gained access to the systemic circulation, a proportion of it is bound to plasma proteins, and the remainder is

distributed throughout the body to other tissues. The extent of this distribution is determined by a number of factors, including the lipid solubility of the drug and the extent of the binding to plasma proteins. Water-soluble, ionized drugs and highly protein bound drugs distribute less extensively. The extent of this distribution is expressed as a volume, *the apparent volume of distribution*, which may far exceed total body volume, indicating concentration of a drug in certain tissues.

Protein binding is important for several reasons. Firstly, because it is only the free, unbound fraction of a drug which is available for interaction with receptor sites for pharmacological action, for tissue distribution, and for biotransformation and subsequent elimination. Secondly, because the amount of drug bound may decrease if the quantity or chemical characteristics of the plasma proteins is affected by hepatic or renal disease. In addition, if two drugs are given concurrently, they compete for the same binding sites and this may result in an increase in the free concentration of one of the drugs: the classical drug interaction of this type is between the oral anti-coagulant warfarin and the non-steroidal, anti-inflammatory drug, phenylbutazone, but rapid redistribution and clearance of the increased free fraction makes toxicity unlikely.

Drug elimination

There are two principal mechanisms by which drugs are eliminated from the body: metabolism within the liver and excretion by the kidneys. Lipid-soluble drugs are not easily excreted in their primary form since, after glomerular filtration, they tend to be reabsorbed by the renal tubule; thus before elimination they need to undergo biotransformation, usually in the liver, to a more water-soluble form (metabolite). In contrast, water-soluble drugs can generally be excreted unchanged by the kidney.

Drugs are metabolized in two phases: phase one consists of metabolic conversion mainly by oxidation by the hepatic microsomal enzymes to a more polar compound; phase two involves conjugation of the drug with another chemical grouping or molecule, usually glucuronic or sulphuric acid. This may also produce an increase in polarity and water solubility, a decrease in pharmacological activity and a greater ease of excretion. Drug metabolism, particularly oxidation, may be affected by severe liver disease, e.g. hepatic cirrhosis, or by substances which either increase (induce) hepatic enzyme activity, such as the anticonvulsants phenytoin, carbamazepine and phenobarbitone, or inhibit it, e.g. the H_2-receptor antagonist cimetidine. Enzyme inhibition and severe liver disease may decrease the rate of elimination of drugs, whereas enzyme induction may accelerate it.

The renal excretion of drugs commonly occurs by glomerular filtration of free drug, e.g. digoxin (p.41) and atenolol (p.47). Active secretion at the proximal tubule may also occur. Impairment of renal function by disease or with advancing age may result in a decrease in the elimination rate of drugs that are excreted by the kidney.

The rate at which a drug is eliminated is called its *clearance*. This is a volume term comparable to creatinine clearance and is defined as the volume of fluid that is completely cleared of drug in unit time. For drugs eliminated by the liver or kidney, the drug clearance may approach hepatic or renal blood flow respectively.

It is customary also to speak of *the elimination half-life of a drug (t$_{1/2}$)*. This is the time required for the plasma concentration to fall by one-half of its original value. The half-life provides useful information for using a drug in clinical practice. Firstly, it helps the physician to determine the most appropriate dosage interval for maintenance treatment, and may influence the method of administration in certain circumstances. Thus, drugs with long half-lives can be given once or twice daily and are useful for long-term therapy; in contrast, drugs with short half-lives must be given more frequently and may require continuous intravenous administration to sustain steady-state plasma concentrations. In general, on commencing administration, it will take about 4–5 half-lives before steady-state concentrations are achieved. This is usually the time for the maximum effect to be reached. Similarly, when toxicity from too high a dose occurs, it will be 4–5 half-lives until the drug is effectively eliminated from the body.

Simple pharmacokinetic information about drugs enables them to be used with maximum efficiency, enabling the best selection, frequency and adjustment of dose.

Drug prescribing

By the time they are available for routine prescription, drugs will have been extensively tested in both animals and man, and, on the basis of these results, will have been granted a licence by the Department of Health and Social Security, indicating that they have satisfied established criteria, particularly in the realm of drug safety. Even so, almost all drugs may produce *adverse effects* in some patients. These fall into two categories: *predictable* from the pharmacological properties of the drug and often the result of excessive pharmacological activity, e.g. postural hypotension in hypersensitive patients treated with certain antihypertensive drugs, and *unpredictable* or idiosyncratic. These latter often take the form of allergic or hypersensitivity responses, are usually unrelated to dose and occur in only a small proportion of patients exposed to the drug. They often present as mild erythematous skin rashes but occasionally may result in life-threatening anaphylactic shock (p.105). Penicillins and sulphonamides frequently produce unpredictable adverse effects.

Elderly patients appear to be particularly likely to experience an adverse effect. This may be partly because many of them suffer from diseases of several systems, and, as a consequence, may be taking a number of different drugs simultaneously. This may also result in an increased possibility of *drug interactions* and decrease drug compliance. These problems may be further compounded by 'over-the-counter' preparations which patients may purchase independently from the pharmacist without prescription—this may now include the non-steroidal anti-inflammatory drug, ibuprofen.

Pregnant women comprise another group where special care in prescribing is necessary. In general, drugs should not be prescribed during pregnancy. In the first trimester, the main risk is that drugs may affect the development of the fetus, e.g. thalidomide produced phocomelia; in the second and third trimesters, drugs may cross the placenta and result in abnormalities at birth, e.g. tetracyclines may result in stained and deformed deciduous teeth, centrally acting drugs may cause neonatal respiratory depression. However, necessary drug therapy should not be withheld.

It follows from the above that patients should only be given drugs for clearly defined therapeutic objectives. When required, the smallest effective dose of the simplest agent should be used. New drugs should only be prescribed if they offer clear benefits over established remedies. When prescribing, drugs already being taken should be reviewed and simplified if possible: drug interactions should be considered. Drugs should be given for specified courses of predetermined length, particularly sedatives like benzodiazepines. However, in certain circumstances, such as hypertension, drug treatment must be continued indefinitiely. When prescriptions are being repeated, the patient should be reviewed from time to time.

Practical aspects of prescribing

Prescriptions should be written legibly and clearly in English and should contain the following information:

1. The patient's full name, address and age.
2. The drug or medicine—preferably by use of the approved or generic name rather than the proprietary name.
3. The strength of tablets, capsules or mixtures. These should be indicated in words and figures (mandatory for controlled drugs).
4. The dose frequency and total quantity to be supplied or the duration of treatment.
5. The prescriber's signature, name and address.
6. The date.

Drug information

The *Dental Practitioners' Formulary* is intended as a pocket reference book for the guidance particularly of dental surgeons. It contains information about the preparations which may be prescribed by dental practitioners on form FP14. It also contains general advice on prescribing and prescription writing. It should be used in conjunction with the *British National Formulary* which is a handbook for medical prescribing. This contains a much wider formulary pertinent for medical prescribing. It is now revised every six months and therefore the information provided is up-to-date.

The dental surgeon requires to use these references in two separate ways: firstly, to obtain information about a limited range of products which he will use in his own dental practice; secondly, it is important that he also seek to identify any other drugs which have been prescribed for the patient by his medical practitioner. This may affect the patient's management for a number of reasons: it may indicate the presence of systemic diseases which could influence dental care, e.g. blood dyscrasias; the drugs may influence the patient's response to treatment, e.g. the anticoagulant drug warfarin may predispose to haemorrhage; centrally acting or anti-hypertensive drugs might affect general anaesthesia; the drugs may interact with the agents which the dentist is intending to use, e.g warfarin and non-steroidal anti-inflammatory drugs. Certain dental drugs may be contra-indicated in patients with certain diseases, e.g. aspirin and non-steroidal anti-inflammatory drugs should not be given to patients with peptic ulcers. These issues are of sufficient potential importance that if the dental practitioner cannot obtain information from the patient and the formularies, he should contact the patient's medical practitioner for clarification.

In addition to the preparations contained in the *Dental Practitioners' Formulary*, dentists may prescribe more widely and in particular, they may use controlled drugs, e.g. narcotic analgesics, though their use is very limited. These preparations are subject to the prescription requirements of the Misuse of Drugs Regulations, 1973.

Prescriptions ordering controlled drugs must be signed and dated by the prescriber and give his address. It must be in the prescriber's own handwriting and contain the information already outlined on p.224. In addition, dental prescriptions must incorporate the words 'for dental treatment only'. Repeat prescriptions are not permitted.

If deciding to use a controlled drug in a particular patient, the dental practitioner must be aware of the prevalence of drug dependence and misuse in Great Britain. The indications for using such a drug should be clearly identified.

20 Hypnotics, sedatives and anxiolytics; analgesics; self-poisoning

There are several groups of drugs which depress the central nervous system. Narcotics, anaesthetics and anticonvulsants are considered elsewhere. Hypnotics are drugs which induce sleep. Sedatives calm the patient without producing sleep although drowsiness may occur. Anxiolytics or tranquillizers relieve excessive anxiety without inducing sleepiness. In practice, there is no clear distinction between these groups of drugs. Most hypnotics act as sedatives if given in small doses and most anxiolytics or sedatives produce sleep if given in larger doses at night. Anxiolytics are sometimes referred to as 'minor tranquillizers' in contrast to 'major tranquillizers' such as chlorpromazine, which are used in psychotic disease such as schizophrenia. This distinction is misleading since the 'major tranquillizers' are sometimes used, in low dose, to relieve anxiety and produce sedation.

All cerebral depressant drugs have the potential danger of producing dependence and tolerance. This leads to difficulty in withdrawing the drug after the patient has been taking it for more than a few weeks. Therefore, hypnotics, sedatives and tranquillizers should not be prescribed indiscriminately. Ideally, they should be given in short courses to alleviate acute symptoms.

Cerebral depressant drugs in large doses cause respiratory depression, which is especially dangerous in patients with advanced chronic respiratory disease. Any cerebral depressant may show exaggerated effects in patients with liver disease, in hypothyroidism and in those already taking drugs with a similar action.

Hypnotics

Insomnia is a symptom, not a disease. Before prescribing a hypnotic an attempt should be made to find the cause of the insomnia: physical illness or discomfort, depression, anxiety, uncongenial environment. Depending on the cause, the appropriate advice and management may not be simply the use of a hypnotic drug.

The most commonly used hypnotics are drugs of the benzodiazepine group, which have, almost completely, replaced the barbiturates. There is now a long list of benzodiazepines, most of which differ very little from each other except in duration of action. In different patients it may be more appropriate to use a long-or short-acting hypnotic. *Nitrazepam* and *flurazepam* have a prolonged action which may give rise to residual hangover effects on the following day and repeated doses tend to be cumulative. *Temazepam* and *triazolam* have a shorter duration and usually cause no hangover effects. *Chloral hydrate* is an effective hypnotic but has the disadvantage of unpleasant taste and gastric irritation. These can be largely avoided by using the compounds dichloralphenazone and triclofos. *Chlormethiazole* is sometimes used as a hypnotic for elderly patients.

Anxiolytics

These drugs should be prescribed only for patients in whom anxiety is a major handicap, interfering with their work or normal life. Where possible, treatment with an anxiolytic drug should be for a short period only, to minimize the dangers of tolerance and dependence.

The drugs most used in the treatment of anxiety are those of the benzodiazepine group. The difference between the many such drugs now available is mainly in duration of action. *Diazepam* and *chlordiazepoxide* have a relatively long duration of action, whereas *oxazepam* and *lorazepam* are shorter-acting.

Barbiturates should no longer be used as tranquillizers or hypnotics. Compared with the benzodiazepines, the barbiturates have a much greater danger of producing habituation and dependence and they are much more dangerous in overdose.

ANALGESICS

The relief of pain is clearly one of the most important and rewarding of therapeutic measures. Pain is commonly associated with anxiety and with other symptoms of the causative disease. The prescriber must take a comprehensive view of the case; frequently some other therapeutic measures are indicated as well as, or sometimes instead of, the prescription of an analgesic. As in any other clinical situation, suitable treatment of pain requires an accurate diagnosis. It must be considered whether the pain would respond to more specific

therapy. Analgesics are frequently employed to relieve pain following dental surgical procedures. In general, analgesics fall into two
groups: non-narcotic analgesics, such as aspirin, and the narcotics,
like morphine.

Non-narcotic analgesics
The main drugs of this group are aspirin and paracetamol. Certain
anti-inflammatory drugs which are particularly used in chronic painful
inflammatory disease such a rheumatoid arthritis are also sometimes
of value as general analgesics in the treatment of pain of moderate
severity.

Aspirin (acetyl-salicyclic acid) is an effective analgesic for headache,
toothache and a wide variety of types of musculoskeletal and somatic
pain. It also has anti-inflammatory properties and is used for this
effect in the rheumatic diseases. Aspirin is antipyretic due to an
action on the hypothalamus. In large doses aspirin causes hypopro-
thrombinaemia. Aspirin reduces platelet aggregation and is used as
a prophylactic in cardiovascular disease.

The usual *analgesic* dose of aspirin for an adult is 600 mg and
nothing is gained from larger single doses. When used for the *anti-
inflammatory* effect in rheumatoid arthritis, larger doses are given. As
well as the plain aspirin tablets, there are tablets containing aspirin
with citric acid and calcium carbonate—dispersible aspirin tablets.

The main adverse effect of aspirin in therapeutic dose is gastric
bleeding from erosions of the gastric mucosa. The majority of normal
subjects lose 3–10 ml daily when taking aspirin regularly. Aspirin
ingestion is a fairly common cause of chronic iron deficiency anaemia
from continuing blood loss. Occasionally massive haemorrhage is
associated with the ingestion of aspirin, particularly if there is an
additional effect from alcohol. Apart from haemorrhage, aspirin may
cause dyspepsia. This is minimized by taking aspirin with meals.
Certain of the proprietary formulations in which aspirin is buffered or
complexed may cause less dyspepsia than plain aspirin but the tendency to gastric bleeding is not eliminated. Enteric coated aspirin
tablets are less liable to cause gastric bleeding and dyspepsia, but
absorption of the aspirin is slow and this type of preparation is
clearly not suitable when rapid, reliable analgesia is required.
Aspirin should not be given to those with a bleeding tendency and
probably should be avoided by patients with disease of the upper
gastrointestinal tract. Allergic reactions, including urticaria and

asthma, occasionally occur, particularly in those with a history of allergy.

The effects of overdose of aspirin include vomiting, tinnitus and deafness. In more severe overdose, coma, convulsions and hyperpyrexia may occur with complicated metabolic changes, the result of a tendency to metabolic acidosis from the accumulation of organic acids and increased catabolism, and a tendency to respiratory alkalosis from stimulation of respiration.

Paracetamol has an analgesic effect similar to that of aspirin. However, it lacks anti-inflammatory properties and so is no substitute for aspirin when the anti-inflammatory action is required. It is a satisfactory alternative to aspirin as a simple analgesic for transient musculo-skeletal pain and has the advantage of not producing gastric bleeding. It is a safe drug in therapeutic dose. In overdose, dangerous, potentially fatal liver damage occurs; this may not become apparent for 4–6 days after poisoning.

Other anti-inflammatory analgesic drugs. Several other anti-inflammatory analgesic drugs, e.g. *ibuprofen* and *naproxen*, can be used as simple analgesics although these are more used in the treatment of rheumatoid arthritis and allied disorders. Although the possibility of gastric haemorrhage is less than with aspirin, the danger is not entirely eliminated.

There are many proprietary preparations consisting of mixtures of analgesics. In general, there is no good evidence of superiority over an adequate dose of a single analgesic and the mixture increases the toxic risk from hypersensitivity or overdose.

Narcotic analgesics
Drugs of this group differ considerably from each other in power and intensity of action, but they have many features in common. Narcotic analgesics relieve pain by actions on the brain, altering the pain threshold and also altering the psychic reaction to the sensation of pain. Narcotic analgesics are appropriate for the relief of visceral pain and severe post-operative or traumatic pain.

The occurrence of addiction is a major problem with the potent narcotic analgesics. Tolerance to morphine is rapidly established and may reach a high degree; an addict may regularly take many times the usual therapeutic dose. Once addiction has occurred, withdrawal of the drug leads to restlessness, anxiety, sweating, lacrimation, cramps, muscular twitching, vomiting, diarrhoea and hallucinations.

The principal actions of narcotic analgesics will be exemplified by listing the actions of morphine. The other narcotic analgesics will then be considered, indicating the major differences from morphine.

Actions of morphine
  CNS
    Analgesia,
    Sedation,
    Respiratory depression,
    Depression of cough reflex,
    Vomiting,
    Miosis,
    Dependence,
    Euphoria.
  Smooth muscle
    Spasm of gastrointestinal muscle causing constipation,
    Spasm of muscle of biliary tract,
    Bronchospasm.

The danger from overdosage of a narcotic analgesic is death from respiratory depression. The potent narcotics are particularly dangerous in patients who already have respiratory insufficiency and in asthmatics because of the additional effect of bronchospasm. They can be dangerous, producing excessive cerebral depressant effects in patients with advanced liver disease or with hypothyroidism.

The narcotic analgesics can be considered in two groups. Firstly, those used in mild to moderate pain and with a relatively low risk of addiction; secondly those used for severe pain and which cause tolerance and dependence.

I.   The first group includes codeine, dihydrocodeine, dextropropoxyphene and pentazocine. Addiction occurs rarely with drugs of this group but is possible.

Codeine is a weak analgesic. Its main use in therapeutics is for cough suppression and for the symptomatic treatment of diarrhoea.

Dihydrocodeine is a more potent analgesic than codeine but less potent than morphine. It is useful for pain of moderate severity which is not adequately controlled by non-narcotic analgesics. It may cause dizziness, and with continued use constipation may be troublesome. It can be given orally or by injection.

Dextropropoxyphene is a relatively weak analgesic, of similar potency to codeine. It has frequently been used in a mixed tablet with *paracetamol* (e.g. *Distalgesic*). The disadvantages of this combination are that overdosage is particularly dangerous and that there is a possibility of drug abuse.

Pentazocine, when given by injection, is more potent than dihydrocodeine but less potent than morphine. It is poorly effective by mouth. Disadvantages include a tendency to hallucinations or nightmares.

II. The second group of narcotic analgesics includes morphine, diamorphine and a group of drugs with similar properties and with high addiction potential.

Morphine is appropriate for the treatment of severe pain of relatively short duration, such as that due to myocardial infarction or after surgery. It is also used in the continuing relief of severe pain in advanced cancer, where the addictive danger is of less significance. However, a potent narcotic analgesic is undesirable in the treatment of recurrent pain in otherwise healthy subjects, such as dysmenorrhoea or headaches, since the real risk of creating a state of addiction would make this therapy unjustified in the great majority of these cases. Morphine is normally given by subcutaneous injection and 10 mg is usually adequate as initial dose. The duration of action of a single injected dose is 4–6 hours. Oral morphine can be used but it is less effective and a relatively larger dose is required. Morphine tends to cause nausea and vomiting and an antiemetic drug, e.g cyclizine, is sometimes given along with morphine to reduce this effect.

Diamorphine (heroin) is a potent analgesic which is more liable to cause euphoria and addiction than morphine but causes less nausea and constipation.

Pethidine is intermediate in analgesic potency between codeine and morphine. It resembles morphine in causing vomiting and addiction but differs in causing less constipation, cough suppression and pupil constriction. It tends to cause atropine-like effects—dry mouth and blurred vision.

Methadone, dextromoramide and *dipipanone* all resemble morphine in actions, although rather less sedating and better absorbed orally.

Buprenorphine is a new analgesic with a duration of action much longer than that of morphine. It can be taken sublingually. It is thought to have less potential for addiction.

Nefopam is a new analgesic, unrelated to the narcotic drugs, and with an unknown mode of action. It has not yet been fully evaluated in oral use.

Antagonism of narcotic drug effects

Naloxone is a competitive antagonist of narcotic drugs. It is used to reverse the respiratory depression produced by an excessive dose of a narcotic drug. When given intravenously, naloxone produces its effect within 1–2 min. Naloxone antagonizes morphine, diamorphine, methadone, pethidine, dihydrocodeine, dextropropoxyphene and pentazocine.

ACUTE DRUG POISONING

During the last twenty years the incidence of self-poisoning has risen considerably in the UK. The treatment of acutely poisoned patients now represents a significant part of the workload of most medical units. Very few such episodes are the result of accidental overdosage and the majority are the consequences of a parasuicidal gesture. A large proportion of such patients ingest *tranquillizers*, *antidepressants* and *hypnotics* whose main action is central nervous system depression and therefore produce unconsciousness. These patients are probably not of relevance to dental practice. However, during the past few years there has been a significant increase in poisoning due to a variety of analgesic agents. Both aspirin and paracetamol are freely available 'over the counter'. In particular, the general public have been educated to believe that paracetamol has fewer side effects than aspirin. However, when combined with the opiate analgesic dextropropoxyphene as *Distalgesic*, overdosage results in a considerable mortality.

Aspirin (salicylate)

Aspirin remains a common household analgesic. The incidence of self-poisoning in adults is therefore frequent. Accidental poisoning in children has been reduced by changes in packaging, however iatrogenic overdosage in children is not uncommon.

Symptoms and signs

Aspirin poisoning is particularly dangerous since the patient who is severely poisoned with marked metabolic chaos is often fully conscious and appears clinically well. In the early phase the patient may complain of tinnitus (ringing in the ears), epigastric pain and breathlessness (due to central stimulation of the respiratory centre). On examination the patient may be sweating and pyrexial. Drowsiness only occurs in the late stages of very severe intoxication and indicates the presence of acidosis. Usually the increase in respiratory rate leads to respiratory alkalosis as the predominant metabolic abnormality.

Treatment

Stomach wash out is followed by efforts to increase urinary salicylate excretion by administration of large amounts of fluid by intravenous infusion and the use of alkali in the form of sodium bicarbonate solution to increase aspirin elimination.

Paracetamol

This drug has gained popularity as a safe alternative to aspirin. However, if ingested in adequate quantity acutely its most significant effect is its potential to produce hepatic necrosis. Children rarely take enough paracetamol either accidentally or as an iatrogenic overdose to give rise to liver damage.

Signs and symptoms

Initially the patient may complain of loss of appetite, nausea and vomiting. Later he may develop abdominal pain and jaundice.

Treatment

In patients diagnosed within 10 hours of ingestion of a significant quantity of paracetamol the use of the specific pharmacological agent *N*-acetylcysteine prevents hepatic damage.

Opiates

Acute opiate poisoning most often occurs in addicts. However, this group of drugs contains a whole range of medium to strong analgesics, all of which may produce characteristic signs of opiate poisoning, viz. respiratory depression, pin-point pupils and coma. Severe respiratory depression can occur even at therapeutic doses in patients who already have respiratory disease, e.g. asthma or chronic bronchitis.

Poisoning is very effectively treated by the administration of the specific pharmacological antagonist *naloxone*.

In dental practice it is important to note that inflammation, excoriation and oedema of nasal and pharyngeal and oral mucosa and circumoral skin may be produced by the habit of 'snorting' not only opiates but also organic solvents and other drugs of abuse.

21 Antimicrobials

GENERAL PRINCIPLES OF ANTIBACTERIAL CHEMOTHERAPY

1. Antibacterials differ from all other groups of drugs in that their present use, by encouraging the emergence of resistant strains, slowly destroys their future value. Overuse hastens this process, exposes the patient to unnecessary risks and wastes money. Antibacterials should never be used to treat fever of unidentified cause or infections due to viruses or fungi.

2. The selection of the correct antibacterial is based on a knowledge of common pathogens present (Table 10). Specimens taken for the bacteriology laboratory before treatment is begun are required to confirm the diagnosis and to identify less common pathogens. *Chemotherapy without microbiology is guesswork.*

3. Bacteriological specimens are often obtained outside laboratory working hours and must then be stored correctly to prevent the death of pathogens or their overgrowth by contaminating bacteria. When pus can be aspirated it should be divided into two sterile containers, one of which is airtight for anaerobic culture, and stored at room temperature. Swabs of pus are less useful because they are often contaminated by skin organisms. Swabs must be stored in transport medium at room temperature. Dry swabs are useless. When symptoms of disseminated infection occur, such as shaking chills (rigors), circulatory impairment or confusion, blood cultures should be taken and stored immediately in an incubator at body temperature.

4. The patient's response to treatment must be interpreted in the light of the bacteriological findings and the source of the specimen. The bacteriology laboratory should be consulted before making a change in treatment.

5. Do not use antibacterials topically on the skin; they are rarely effective, often cause sensitivity reactions and can lead to the rapid development of bacterial resistance.

6. The need to continue treatment after symptoms have resolved must be impressed upon the patient. After serious infections, take test-of-cure specimens.

Table 10. Pathogens responsible for common dental infections and recommended antibacterial agents.

Clinical infection	Common pathogens	First choice treatment	Alternative in case of drug allergy	Rare pathogens	First choice	Alternative
Acute necrotizing ulcerative gingivitis	Mixed aerobic (viridans streptococcus) and anaerobic species	Benzyl penicillin	Erythromycin	Penicillin-resistant Bacteroides	Metronidazole	Clindamycin
Apical abscess	Anaerobic streptococci; fusobacteria; penicillin-sensitive bacteroides sp.	Benzyl penicillin				
Tonsillitis	*Streptococcus pyogenes*	Benzyl penicillin	Erythromycin			
Deep space infections including Ludwig's angina	Mixed aerobic and penicillin-sensitive anaerobic species	Benzyl penicillin	Erythromycin	(a) Penicillin-resistant Bacteroides	Metronidazole	Clindamycin
				(b) *Staphylococcus aureus**	Flucloxacillin	
Paranasal sinusitis	*Streptococcus pneumoniae; Haemophilus influenzae*	Amoxycillin	Co-trimoxazole			

* Staphylococcal infection should be suspected when there is a primary lesion on the overlying skin

7. Non-proprietary mixtures of antibacterial drugs are justified for severe infections when no single agent covers the range of potential pathogens, otherwise co-trimoxazole provides the only example of rational combination chemotherapy (p.240).

REASONS FOR FAILURE OF ANTIBACTERIAL THERAPY

1. The symptoms are not due to bacterial infection. Common causes of 'failure' are infections due to viruses, fungi or *Mycobacterium tuberculosis*, all of which are resistant to standard antibacterials. The major non-infective causes of pyrexia are tumours, especially lymphomas, and connective tissue diseases, especially giant cell arteritis and polyarteritis nodosa.
2. Failure by the patient to take full doses, to complete the full course of therapy, or to absorb enough from the gut. Serious infection should be treated with parenteral antibiotic for at least the first 48–72 hours.
3. The presence of a collection of pus which requires surgical drainage. This may not be obvious clinically. Occult foci in the head and neck include the deep tissue spaces and paranasal sinuses and, in the abdomen, spaces under the diaphragm or under the liver. Osteomyelitis (p.18) may also require drainage and is unlikely to begin to improve until completion of the first week of treatment.
4. The infecting bacterium is resistant to the treatment given. A change of treatment should be directed at potential pathogens which are resistant to first line treatment (Table 10). If the organism has not been identified, take appropriate cultures before changing therapy.

COMPLICATIONS OF ANTIBACTERIAL TREATMENT

Dose-related side effects and idiosyncrasy
Fortunately most dose-related antibacterial side-effects occur only in patients who have some predisposing factor (idiosyncrasy). Prescribers should restrict the number of drugs which they use regularly and be aware of all potential idiosyncrasies to each.

Hypersensitivity reactions
These range from transitory rashes to fatal anaphylactic shock (p.105). Patients must be asked about previous drug reactions but

non-allergic side effects, such as nausea or diarrhoea, must be differentiated from true allergy. About 50% of patients who are allergic
to the penicillins also react to the cephalosporins and vice versa but
serious reactions are rare. If a drug must be used in a patient
with a history of allergy to it, a small test dose can be given in an
intensive care unit with full resuscitation facilities.

Gastrointestinal side effects, including antibiotic-associated colitis (AAC)

Mild nausea and diarrhoea are common side effects of many antibacterials and do not require a change in therapy. AAC, also known as
pseudomembranous colitis, is a serious disease caused by a toxin of
Clostridium difficile. This anaerobe colonizes the bowel of patients
who are receiving antibacterial drugs, especially clindamycin and
ampicillin, but AAC has been associated with most antibacterials. The
presenting symptoms are profuse, watery or bloody diarrhoea, and
abdominal pain. Severe cases show systemic signs of toxaemia and
can be fatal. When the diagnosis is suspected antibacterial treatment
should be stopped; the diagnosis should be confirmed by sigmoidoscopy and by isolation of toxin from the stools. Paradoxically, AAC
responds dramatically to either of two oral antibacterial drugs:
vancomycin or metronidazole. Anti-diarrhoeal drugs are absolutely
contraindicated because they increase the risk of systemic toxaemia.

Antibiotic-associated superinfection

Superinfection is defined as secondary infection by resistant organisms during antibacterial treatment: oropharyngeal candidosis is a
common example, particularly during tetracycline therapy.

DRUGS RECOMMENDED FOR USE IN DENTAL INFECTIONS

Penicillins

Toxic effects

Dose-related and idiosyncratic. These drugs are excreted mainly by
the kidney. Dangerous accumulation leading to convulsions occurs
if doses are not reduced in severe renal failure.

Ampicillin is poorly absorbed and commonly causes gastrointestinal side effects; amoxycillin is better tolerated and probably more effective. Ampicillin and amoxycillin cause florid rashes in patients with glandular fever (p.288) and lymphatic tumours (the lymphatic leukaemias and lymphomas) and if given in unreduced doses to patients with severe renal failure.

Hypersensitivity reactions. These are rare but can be serious. They include the classical allergic reactions such as urticaria, angioneurotic oedema or asthma as well as more organ-specific reactions such as acute interstitial nephritis, bone marrow suppression or haemolytic anaemia. Patients with allergy to one penicillin will be allergic to all penicillins and possibly to cephalosporins as well.

Table 11   Penicillins for use in dental infection.

	Mode of administration	Activity against important dental pathogens
Benzyl penicillin Phenoxymethyl penicillin	Intramuscular/intravenous. oral	Streptococci Oral anaerobes except Bacteroides sp.
Cloxacillin	Intramuscular/intravenous/ oral	*Staphylococcus aureus*
Ampicillin Amoxycillin	Intramuscular/intravenous/ oral	Streptococci *Haemophilus influenzae*

Erythromycin

Side effects. Erythromycin injections are highly irritant. They should therefore be given by slow intravenous infusion and never by intramuscular injection.

Erythromycin causes gastrointestinal side effects more frequently than the penicillins and occasionally causes rashes but not serious hypersensitivity reactions.

Use in dental infections. The many brands of erythromycin are essentially similar, except that the estolate form may cause idiosyncratic

240

Chapter 21

hepatotoxicity and is therefore contraindicated in patients with liver disease. Erythromycin is active against streptococci, *Staphylococcus aureus*, some *Haemophilus influenzae* and anaerobic organisms. However, widespread use results in drug resistance, particularly by *Staphylococcus aureus* or *Haemophilus influenzae*. Erythromycin is less effective than co-trimoxazole for Haemophilus infections. Its main use is as an alternative to penicillin in allergic patients.

Co-trimoxazole
Co-trimoxazole is a mixture of trimethoprim with the sulphonamide sulphamethoxazole. Both drugs inhibit bacterial DNA synthesis by interfering with folate metabolism. The major reason for combining the two agents was to kill bacteria that had become resistant to either component. This has always been a controversial issue and trimethoprim is now marketed as a single agent. Use of trimethroprim alone has not resulted in increased resistance amongst urinary pathogens but there is still reason to believe that it should not be used alone for Haemophilus infections. The use of co-trimoxazole for appropriate dental infections is therefore recommended.

Side effects are of two kinds:
1. *Dose-related and idiosyncratic*
   Sulphamethoxazole does not affect human folate metabolism. Trimethroprim has a negligible effect in normal people but may be harmful in patients with vitamin B_{12} or folic acid deficiency, including pregnant women, and, because of drug accumulation, in severe renal failure.
2. *Hypersensitivity*
   Rashes occur in sulphonamide-sensitive patients. The Stevens–Johnson syndrome is a rare but potentially fatal complication of sulphamethoxazole therapy. The major symptoms are severe blistering of the skin and ulceration of mucous membranes.
   In addition to the dose-related antihaemopoietic effect of trimethoprim, sulphamethoxazole very rarely causes agranulocytosis or aplastic anaemia in hypersensitive patients.

Use in dental infections. Co-trimoxazole is available in oral and intravenous forms. It is less effecive than penicillins or erythromycin for staphylococcal infections and does not have clinically useful activity against anaerobic organisms. It is an alternative to amoxycillin for the treatment of middle ear and paranasal sinus infections and should be used as a first choice in infections due to amoxycillin-resistant *Haemophilus influenzae.*

Metronidazole
Metronidazole acts only against anaerobic species.

Side effects. Dose-related: none with antibacterial dosages. Idiosyncratic: metronidazole inhibits the metabolism of alcohol causing accumulation of acetaldehyde, the metabolite responsible for 'hangovers'.

Use in dental infections. Metronidazole should be used for the treatment of infections due to Bacteroides sp. Metronidazole and penicillin should be combined empirically for severe infections of the oropharyngeal tissue spaces when signs of systemic toxaemia are present. For most infections it is reasonable to use penicillin alone because most oral anaerobes are penicillin-sensitive.

Gentamicin
The use of gentamicin in dental practice is limited to the prophylaxis of endocarditis (p.38); at these dosages it has no important side effects. The risk of dose-related renal impairment, deafness and vestibular damage increases progressively as therapy is increased beyond three days.

Clindamycin
Clindamycin is available in oral and parenteral forms.

Clindamycin has excellent activity against streptococci, *Staphylococcus aureus* and all anaerobic organisms. Its use is limited by its propensity for causing antibiotic-associated colitis (p.238) but it is a useful reserve drug for the oral treatment of staphylococcal infection in patients with penicillin allergy.

Other antibacterials available for dental practice
These drugs are discussed briefly because it is our belief that they are rarely required in current dental practice.

Cephalosporins (cephalexin, cephradine)
These are more expensive than the penicillins, have essentially the same range of activity, but are less effective against dental pathogens. They should not be used for treating Haemophilus infections.

Cephalosporins have the same side effects as penicillins and should not be used in penicillin-allergic patients.

Anti-fungal agents

Nystatin
Nystatin is not absorbed from the gut and is used for the topical treatment of mucosal candidosis. Oral candidosis requires the application of nystatin solution by dropper; this is effective for localized infection. Nystatin has no important side effects.

Amphotericin
Amphotericin is not absorbed from the gut; amphotericin lozenges are particularly useful for treating generalized oral candidosis and do not have important side effects. Intravenously administered amphotericin is highly nephrotoxic but remains the only effective treatment for most systemic fungal infections.

Imidazoles
This large group of drugs includes a number of topical agents as well as one intravenous formulation (miconazole) and ketoconazole which is absorbed from the gut. The imidazoles have replaced older drugs for the treatment of fungal infections of the skin, nails and vagina but do not have significant advantages over nystatin or amphotericin for oral candidosis. They are also much more expensive.

If oral candidosis fails to respond to nystatin or amphotericin, a deficiency of cell-mediated immunity should be suspected and the patient referred to hospital. Patients who develop oral candidosis during cytotoxic chemotherapy require careful evaluation for the presence of deep infection of the pharynx or oesophagus which can only be treated with systemic amphotericin.

Antiviral agents
Antiviral chemotherapy is a rapidly expanding field and the clinician is now being faced with a choice of drugs for the treatment of common viral infections. It is vital to keep a clear picture of the aims and limitatons of antiviral therapy. The agents which are currently available are effective aginst herpes simplex virus types 1 and 2 (the

cause respectively of oral and genital herpes infection) and moderately effective against varicella zoster (the cause of chickenpox and herpes zoster [shingles]).

These drugs now make a major contribution to the treatment of herpes infections in immunocompromised patients. People with normal immunity have self-limiting infections and there is scant evidence for significant benefit from expensive drug therapy. The real problem in this group is with recurrent mucocutaneous herpes simplex infection.

Idoxuridine
Only available for topical use as a 5% paint. Contact with mucous membranes is painful and it is not as effective as acyclovir.

Acyclovir
Available as a cream (not to be confused with the ointment which is exclusively used for eye infections), as tablets or as intravenous infusion. All these formulations reduce the duration of symptoms of oral herpes simplex by about 24 hours provided the treatment is started within 48 hours of onset. Acyclovir does not prevent recurrent attacks which are due to persistence of herpes simplex within nerve ganglia where the virus is protected from the drug. All the formulations are expensive and should be reserved mainly for treating severe infections in patients with impaired immunity. Normal people with frequent, severe recurrences of oral herpes may benefit from keeping a supply of acyclovir cream at home to use at the first onset of symptoms. Continuous, prophylactic use of acyclovir is not justified in this group.

Acyclovir cream has no important side effects.

Inosine pranobex
The mode of action of this drug is not clear. it may act both as an antiviral agent and as a stimulator of T-lymphocytes. It has recently been licensed in the UK for the treatment of herpes simplex infection and there is some evidence that it reduces the rate of recurrent attacks but there are as yet no trials comparing it with acyclovir.

Other antiviral agents will continue to appear on the market; the clinician must continually question whether the symptomatic benefit, which should be greater than evidence of 'reduced duration of viral shedding', justifies their considerable expense.

22 Social implications of health

Smoking

Tobacco has been smoked in one form or another since Elizabethan times, but it is only very recently that the health implications, particularly of cigarette smoking, have been realized. It was not until the 1950s that careful epidemiological research demonstrated a clear association between smoking and lung cancer. More recently, associations with other conditions such as chronic obstructive lung disease, coronary heart disease, peripheral vascular disease, some abnormalities of pregnancy and some non-pulmonary forms of cancer, e.g. mouth, larynx, oesophagus, pancreas and bladder, have been recognized.

Because cigarette smoking is so prevalent, the implications for health care and economics are considerable. For instance, 15–20% of all deaths in the UK are directly related to smoking. It is estimated that 50 million working days are lost each year in the UK as a result of smoking-related illness and that it costs 6 million per year to pay the medical and nursing staff to treat these conditions in Scotland alone.

Fortunately, over the past 5–10 years there has been a slight reduction in tobacco consumption although this reduction is largely due to a change in the smoking habits of men, and not of women.

Smoking and lung cancer

The link between smoking and the development of bronchial carcinoma is well established. The risk increases proportionately with:
1. The number of cigarettes smoked per day,
2. The number of years indulging in cigarette smoking (particularly if smoking began early in life),
3. The tar content of cigarettes.

Bronchial carcinoma is one of the commonest single causes of death in the western world and the vast majority of cases can be directly attributed to cigarette smoking. There have been a few recent reports of increases in the incidence of bronchial carcinoma in the non-smoking spouses of cigarette smokers suggesting that 'passive' smoking may not be entirely harmless. A person who smokes more than 25 cigarettes per day will carry 30–40 times the risk of dying from bronchial carcinoma compared to a non-smoker. Not all long-term heavy smokers develop bronchial carcinoma, however, and there are obviously other factors which determine a patient's susceptibility to the disease.

Smoking and chronic obstructive lung disease
Cigarette smoking has been shown to produce over-secretion of bronchial mucus, interference with clearance of mucus from airways and to increase susceptibility to respiratory infection. These effects, plus a possible toxic effect on lung tissue, cause a gradual deterioration in lung function over the years. In some smokers this deterioration is slight but in others it can be great, leading to respiratory failure and death.

A person smoking more than 25 cigarettes per day has 25 times the risk of dying from chronic obstructive lung disease compared to a non-smoker. There are, however, other factors responsible for the development of this condition, such as air pollution, low social class, occupation and a history of chest disease in childhood.

Smoking and heart disease
Coronary heart disease is one of the commonest diseases in the western world. Although a multifactorinal condition, cigarette smoking is one of the three major risk factors, the others being hypertension and a raised serum cholesterol. Lesser risk factors include age, obesity, physical inactivity and genetic factors.

Necropsy studies have shown more advanced coronary artery narrowing in smokers. It has also been shown that smokers are more likely to develop intravascular occlusive thrombi. The nicotine in tobacco has been shown to be able to increase the heart's susceptibility to rhythm disorders.

Cigarette smokers are therefore more prone to angina, myocardial infarction and sudden cardiac death than non-smokers.

Smoking and peripheral vascular disease
Narrowing of peripheral arteries and arterioles appears to be increased in smokers. The resulting reduction in blood supply can lead to

pain in the limbs during exercise (intermittent claudication). In more severe cases, the limb pain can occur at rest, leading eventually to tissue necrosis or gangrene. More than 90% of patients suffering from peripheral vascular disease have been heavy smokers (more than 20 cigarettes/day) for 20 years or more and the condition rarely occurs in non-smokers.

Arterial aneurysm and stroke are also commoner in cigarette smokers. Where vascular disease has been treated by implantation of grafts, it has become clear that the grafts are more likely to occlude if the patient continues to smoke after surgery.

Smoking and reproduction
It appears that cigarette-smoking women are more likely to be sub-fertile or infertile suggesting that smoking affects ovarian function. The fact that cigarette smokers have an earlier menopause than non-smokers also supports this.

During pregnancy, smoking increases the risk of antepartum haemorrhages and spontaneous abortion but it reduces the incidence of toxaemia. The babies of smokers tend to be 0.25 kg lighter than the babies of non-smokers and have a slightly increased perinatal mortality.

The risk of myocardial infarction and stroke are increased by smoking and the contraceptive pill. When the contraceptive pill and smoking are combined, especially in women over 35 years, the risk of developing either of these conditions appears to be very much increased to 10–15 times normal.

Because most of the health risks that are associated with cigarette smoking are relatively untreatable, smoking prevention is obviously the most effective means of reducing the incidence of these risks.

Low tar cigarettes have been introduced but, although they confer some benefit with regard to development of bronchial carcinoma or chronic obstructive lung disease, the effects in pregnancy or in development of coronary heart disease remain unchanged.

Health education has helped reduce tobacco consumption, particularly in men, and the reports from the Royal College of Physicians have played a major part. The Health Education Council (HEC) and Action on Smoking and Health (ASH) continue to try to reduce cigarette consumption by advertising campaigns directed towards specific groups of people, education of children, etc.

Effective legislation reducing cigarette advertising and introducing punitive taxation on tobacco products has also helped to some extent.

Obesity

Obesity is common in affluent socities and is associated with abnormal accumulation of fat in the adipose tissue throughout the body. It carries excess mortality, e.g. by predisposing to diabetes mellitus (p.129) and its consequences.

Genetic and environmental factors are both important in its aetiology and women are more prone to obesity than men and especially so after pregnancy or at the menopause. Consuming more calories than is necessary to match energy output results in weight gain, especially below a certain level of exercise. Obese individuals are often psychologically upset but cause and effect are difficult to distinguish. Skin-fold thickness over the triceps muscle is useful in the clinical assessment of the degree of obesity, as are weight/height charts.

Complications of obesity include osteoarthritis of the main weight-bearing joints (lumbar, spine, hips and knees, p.156), proneness to accidents, herniae (p.122), varicose veins, bronchitis from mechanical interference with respiration, increased peri-operative morbidity and mortality, and chronic skin infection between fat folds (intertrigo), e.g. under the breasts. Hyperlipidaemia, gall-stones, diabetes mellitus, gout, cardiovascular disorders and decreased life-expectancy are other noted complications.

No single factor causes obesity, but as it always represents the accumulation of more energy than the body requires, it is clear that successful weight reduction requires decreased food intake, increased energy expenditure, or both. Treatment comprises patient education and support, e.g. 'Weight Watchers' groups, supervised weight-reducing diet, sometimes anorectic drugs, and increased exercise. Successful long-term weight reduction is seldom achieved. In intractable cases of severe obesity, wiring of the jaws to limit eating or small intestinal bypass operations to restrict food absorption help a select minority.

Dependence on drugs and alcohol

Drug dependence may be psychological or physical. Psychological dependence implies a compulsion to repeat taking the drug to experience its effects or to avoid the effects of its withdrawal. Physical dependence refers to the development of physical disturbance when the drug is withdrawn.

There is a complex relationship between dependence on drugs and alcohol and psychiatric disorders. Individuals with personality disorders and neurotic illnesses will obtain symptomatic relief from alcohol and certain drugs. This results in these people being particularly vulnerable to becoming dependent on alcohol and drugs. In contrast, certain psychiatric conditions arise as a result of drug or alcohol dependence.

Alcoholism is a widespread problem resulting in considerable social and economic problems and personal misery. Long-term over-indulgence in alcohol may result in serious personality deterioration and dementia. Delirium tremens is an acute confusional state which usually develops in relation to alcohol withdrawal. Epileptic fits (p.179) may also occur in relation to alcohol withdrawal. Alcohol abuse is also the commonest cause of liver cirrhosis (p.124).

Dependence on prescribed drugs such as barbiturates and benzodiazepines is relatively common. Barbiturate dependence may result in a state of chronic intoxication with slurring of speech and ataxia similar to alcohol intoxication. Withdrawal of barbiturates results in both psychological and physical symptoms, including epileptic fits.

Although dependence on opiates such as morphine and diamorphine is increasing, it is still considerably less common than dependence on alcohol and prescribed drugs. Opiate dependence attracts much more attention because of the legal implications and associated lifestyle and the premature death of a number of previously fit young people from overdose, sepsis and hepatitis. Opiates produce both physical and psychological dependence and the withdrawal syndrome is very unpleasant but not as dangerous as barbiturate withdrawal.

Dental aspects of pregnancy
All female patients of reproductive age should be asked about the possibility of pregnancy prior to giving dental treatment. Pregnancy is the ideal time for advice to the mother on the importance of dental hygiene, but elective dental treatment is best deferred until after the baby is born. Treatment should still be given to relieve pain, to treat infection or to stop a disease getting worse. An awareness of the effects of drugs on the fetus and the baby is necessary when dental treatment of the pregnant or nursing mother is undertaken. Regardless of the stage of pregnancy, therefore, it is important to contact the patient's obstetrician before starting treatment.

Necessary treatment should preferably be postponed until after the first trimester because of possible teratogenic effects of some drugs. Stress to the mother should also be avoided at all times in order to avoid premature labour and reassurance is therefore important. In the second half of pregnancy, the patient should not be put in a supine posture. This may cause the supine hypotensive syndrome which is characterized by tachycardia, pallor and faintness due to compression of the inferior vena cava by the uterus. All patients should therefore be treated in the left lateral position.

Radiographs are best avoided to prevent irradiation of the fetus. If they are essential, protective aprons should be used to shield the mother's abdomen.

Almost all drugs cross the placenta and, in nursing mothers, appear in breast milk. Therefore, only drugs known to be safe in pregnancy should be used, particularly in the first trimester. Centrally acting drugs such as barbiturates and benzodiazepines should be avoided as they also affect the fetus.

Nitrous oxide (N_2O) in high concentration can harm the fetus and lead to anoxia. Short-term use of low concentrations of N_2O for dental treatment is reported to be safe. Local anaesthetics are also safe, but care should be taken to avoid their intravascular injection. Vasoconstrictor drugs should be avoided as they may cross the placenta and affect the fetal circulation. Felypressin seems less likely to initiate uterine contraction than was formerly feared. The commonly used antibiotics (p.238) are safe when used for short periods, especially after the first trimester.

The dental treatment of nursing mothers is less of a problem, but it must be remembered that drugs are secreted in the breast milk and so may affect the baby.

Contraception

Effective contraception has transformed the role of women in society, and the widespread use of oral contraceptives testifies to their popularity. Pregnancy can now be avoided or planned to fit in with a woman's domestic needs or her career.

Effectiveness of currently available methods

Douching, withdrawal, rhythm and spermicides are all unreliable methods.

Condom, cap (or diaphragm) and a progesterone-only pill are reliable if correctly used (pregnancy rate 2–3 per 100 woman years [WY]).

Intrauterine devices are reliable (1.5–3.0 per 100 WY).

Combined oestrogen-progestogen pills are very reliable if correctly used (0.1 – 0.4/100 WY).

Sterilization or vasectomy is very reliable (< 0.5/100 WY).

Post-coital (morning after) contraception using a high-dose combined pill for two days, or an emergency IUD fitting, have only a 1% failure.

Barrier methods
The condom (or sheath) is still used almost as much as the combined pill. It is a safe method if carefully used and along with spermicidal jelly. It also helps to protect those at risk from venereal disease (p.252).

The diaphragm (or cap) is effective in a well-motivated woman. It must be inserted before intercourse with spermicidal jelly and left for some hours afterwards before removal for cleaning and careful storage.

Combined oestrogen–progestogen pills
These are generally convenient and effective, but they are potent drugs and present an unacceptable risk to women with certain medical or social circumstances. They work by inhibiting ovulation, replacing the normal hormone cycle. They also alter the endometrium making it unfavourable for implantation, and adversely affect the cervical mucus and tubal motility.

The combined pill is taken for 21 days, followed by a pill-free week when a withdrawal bleed or period is expected to occur. With the newer lower dose pills it is even more important that they be taken at the same time each day for maximum effect.

There are well-recognized risks to women taking the combined pill but they can be minimized by careful prescribing and follow-up. The risk of DVT or pulmonary thromboembolism is associated with the oestrogen component and this risk is reduced by using not more than 50 μg per day of oestrogen, and excluding those with a history of such problems from using the combined pill. The pill should be stopped six weeks prior to any operation that will entail prolonged immobilization.

The risk of cardiovascular complications such as myocardial infarction, stroke or hypertension may be related to the doses of both oestrogen and progestogen, and a rising blood pressure or headaches while on the combined pill is an indication for stopping it. These risks are strongly related to cigarette smoking, obesity, age (the combined pill should preferably not be used beyond the age of 35 years), and diseases such as diabetes mellitus, hypertension, and familial hyperlipidaemia. These risks are minimized by keeping to as low a dose of each component as is consistent with effective contraception. Social circumstances often dictate that the risks of unwanted pregnancy often outweigh these medical hazards.

The use of oral contraceptives appears to predispose to candidosis of the vulva and vagina (p.104) and this is often resistant to treatment. In some women they also cause ureteric dilatation (similar to that during pregnancy) and so may predispose to coliform infections of the urinary tract.

There is recent controversy concerning 'the pill' and cancer. The present concensus is that the combined pill does not increase the risk of breast cancer, may rarely induce liver tumours, and may slightly increase the risk of cervical cancer. The effects of the latter can be greatly reduced by regular cervical cytological screening.

Drug interactions
Certain drugs can reduce the contraceptive effect of 'the pill' through liver enzyme induction (p.221), e.g. rifampicin, phenytoin and carbamazepine rarely and some antibiotics; conversely, the pill can adversely affect the treatment of some diseases such as diabetes mellitus with insulin or oral hypoglycaemic drugs, depression with tricyclic antidepressants, hypertension with drug treatment or thromboembolic states treated with warfarin. The effects of theophylline, prednisolone and diazepam may be enhanced because of decreased metabolism.

In most women the pill causes no problems, and as long as breast, cervical cytology and blood pressure checks are carried out regularly, the combined pill may be used safely throughout the whole reproductive life.

Progestogen-only pills
These are used for women for whom the combined pill is contraindicated, e.g. during breast feeding, or who develop side effects on it.

They are taken daily with no pill-free interval in the month. They are not so effective as the combined pill and may cause an irregular menstrual pattern. They work by altering the cervical mucus making it unfavourable for sperm penetration, and the endometrium unfavourable for implantation.

Injectable progestogen
The injectable long-acting progestogen medroxyprogesterone acetate (*Depo-Provera*), which is given every three months, is advised for certain restricted situations such as covering a short-term crisis, or for those for whom there is no suitable alternative. Apart from giving a disturbed menstrual bleeding pattern, its main disadvantage is an uncertain delay in the return of fertility after it is stopped. Long-term follow-up research for this method is still in progress.

Intrauterine devices
These are made of plastic and are designed in various shapes to fit the uterine cavity. Many bear a coil of copper wire which enhances their efficacy. They act by altering the endometrium, making it unfavourable for implantation. They are used as an alternative to the combined pill and can be used until the menopause is complete. They are not recommended for nullipara because of the slight risk of pelvic infection which could lead to persistent infertility.

The pregnancy rate is low when the device is fitted by an experienced doctor. The copper-bearing devices are small and designed to minimize the chance of uterine perforation, and careful selection of patients reduces the chance of pelvic infection. The patient should be examined annually for two or three years depending on the recommended life of the particular IUD used. Most women using an IUD have no significant side effects.

Venereal disease
Venereal diseases are almost invariably contracted during sexual intercourse. Gonorrhoea and other forms of urethritis are common in Britain because of changing social attitudes to sexual intercourse, but syphilis is now rare. The widespread use of oral contraception in preference to barrier methods (p.250) encourages the spread of gonococcal and non-specific urethritis.

Gonorrhoea

Causal organism. Gonococcus (*Neisseria gonorrhoea*).

Clinical features. The incidence of gonorrhoea has risen markedly in recent years, the 16–24 yr age groups being most often affected. Infection is characterized by:
1. Purulent urethral discharge (both sexes) 4–10 days after contact.
2. Vaginal discharge in the female.
3. Dysuria and frequency of micturition (both sexes).

Complications include spread of infection to the eye (conjunctivitis) and the joints (gonococcal arthritis). In females spread up the genital tract may cause inflammation of the fallopian tubes (salpingitis) with abdominal pain and fever. Sterility may be a late complication of salpingitis. Affected males may get prostatitis or, as a late complication, stricture of the urethra.

Treatment. Most cases respond rapidly to penicillin. If the organisms are resistant to this drug, or if the patient is allergic to penicillin alternative treatment should be with either co-trimoxazole or spectinomycin.

Note. Many other infections can be transmitted by sexual contact. The more important of these are the following: chlamydial infection, herpes simplex, candidosis, trichomonal infection, genital warts, viral hepatitis type 'B' and the AIDS syndrome.

Syphilis
A contagious venereal disease infection carried by the spirochaete *Treponema pallidum*. Since the advent of penicillin the disease has declined but it is still relatively common, particularly amongst male homosexuals. The natural history of the disease is divided into three stages:

Primary stage. This is characterized by the appearance of a painless superficial ulcer (*chancre*) at the site of inoculation together with enlargement of the regional lymph nodes, one to eight weeks after infection. The chancre is usually on the genitals but *it may be found in the mouth* or in the ano-rectal region. This primary lesion is *highly infective*. It heals in about two to three weeks.

Secondary stage. This stage occurs three to six weeks after the appearance of the chancre. There is fever and generalized lympha-denopathy. A copper-coloured rash appears on the skin. Warty lesions (condylomata) may also occur in the perineum and around the mouth. 'Snail track' ulcers are found on the oral mucosa. All these lesions are *highly infective*. They will fade even in the untreated patient. Untreated, the disease will inevitably progress to the tertiary stage.

Tertiary stage. This may occur at any time, even many years after the secondary stage, giving rise to:
1. Small nodular non-infective granulomata (gummata) which may appear in the skin, mouth or in any internal site. These gummata often break down to form chronic ulcers.
2. Central nervous system involvement.
3. Aortitis, causing aortic incompetence and, in some cases, aortic aneurysm may result.

Diagnosis. This may be confirmed by the isolation of the sphirochaetes from lesions in the primary and secondary stages of the disease, or by specific serological tests (TPHA and TPI tests).

Treatment. 600 000–900 000 units of procaine penicillin daily for 10–21 days, depending on the stage of the disease.

Note. Treatment, follow-up and contact tracing should be under the supervision of a specialist in sexually transmitted diseases.

23   Disorders of the skin and
mucous membranes

Cutaneous diseases

Examination of skin includes the assessment of the mucous membranes of the mouth and genitalia, together with the nails and the hair. The lesions of skin diseases are defined as primary or secondary and are described below:

Primary lesions

Macule. Circumscribed discoloured flat areas of varying shapes, e.g. freckles, vitiligo.

Papule. Raised localized firm lesions up to 5 mm in diameter, e.g. acne, folliculitis.

Plaque. Confluence of raised papular lesions, e.g. psoriasis.

Telangiectasia. Dilated capillaries visible on the skin.

Erythema. Redness due to vasodilatation caused by inflammation.

Weal. Transient ill-defined raised lesions, e.g. urticaria.

Vesicle. Small elevated collections of fluid, e.g. herpes simplex.

Bullae. Larger vesicles more than 5 mm in diameter containing fluid, e.g. impetigo, pemphigoid.

Purpura. Non-compressible area of red blood cells within the skin, e.g. bleeding disorders.

Pustule. Pocket or collection of pus, i.e. small abscess.

Nodule. Circumscribed solid palpable lesion deep in the skin, e.g. erythema nodosum.

Tumour. Larger nodule or palpable mass in the skin.

Secondary lesions

Scale. Thickened loosely detachable superficial layers of skin, e.g. fungus, psoriasis.

Crust. Collection of dried exudate containing bacteria and leucocytes.

Ulcer. Irregularly shaped excavations with loss of epidermis and dermis.

Lichenification. Thickening of epidermis with accentuation of skin lines.

Erosions. Superficial ulcerations of mucous membrane.

Affections of the lips and oral cavity

Cheilitis
An acute inflammation of the lips causing severe dryness, fissuring and discomfort. The common causes are exposure to sunlight, severe cold and allergic reaction to certain foods or antibiotic therapy.
   (A rare cause is pellagra, due to niacin deficiency, p.168.)

Angular stomatitis
This is caused by ill-fitting dentures, oral candidosis and anaemia.

Herpes simplex
This is caused by herpes simplex virus type I. Consists of a group of vesicles at the mucocutaneous junction of the mouth; painful and ulcerated with regional lymphadenopathy. The lesion develops in a day or two and persists for three to six days. Reactivation of virus gives rise to recurrent episodes. Antiviral agents such as idoxuridine and acyclovir are beneficial if used in the pre-eruptive phase. During the active phase, topical povidone-iodine solution is useful as a

symptomatic measure. The oral lesions tend to clear within about a week.

Erythema multiforme
This is an erythematous blistering condition characterized by 'target lesions' affecting the skin and mucous membrane of mouth and eyes. The oral blisters rupture easily producing erosions and ulceration. The aetiology is usually viral, bacterial or due to drugs. The severe type of erythema multiforme may require systemic steroid therapy.

Hand, foot and mouth disease
This is caused by Coxsackie A virus producing vesiculation and ulceration of the oral cavity associated with tiny vesicles on the hands, fingers and soles of the feet. Outbreaks of the viral infection occur in children. Antiviral agents are not effective.

Trigeminal herpes zoster
The muco-cutaneous lesions are unilateral and affect the fifth cranial nerve causing vesicles in the mouth and cheek. This is a painful condition with paraesthesiae and sensory disturbances on the affected side. Symptomatic treatment with analgesics or amitriptyline is needed. Antiviral drugs are also sometimes used.

Aphthous ulceration
Recurrent ulcers occur on the buccal mucosa and tongue which can be painful and persistent. Sometimes the ulcers are associated with folate or vitamin B_{12} deficiency or underlying gastrointestinal disorders such as coeliac disease. The ulcers may heal by scarring. Hydrocortisone pellets may help in healing the ulcer. Chlorhexidine mouth washes or tetracycline rinses are effective measures. Triamcinalone acetonide in orabase and benzydamine oral rinse may be useful applications.

Leukoplakia
Leukoplakia is a chronic whitish lesion which appears on the buccal mucosa and the lip margin due to prolonged irritation. Tobacco smoking or chewing or pipe smoking may cause the lesions. Only a small number of these patients develop malignant transformation. Histological study of the lesions is essential. Leukoplakia does not imply malignant change.

Geographical tongue

In *'geographical tongue'* the dorsal aspect usually shows sharply marginated smooth red areas. Papillary atrophy is seen. The aetiology is unknown. It is asymptomatic.

Lichen planus

Oral lesions are characterized by a network of white striae sharply demarcated on the buccal mucosa. These lesions are mostly asymptomatic. At times they can be atrophic with thinning and erosions, causing pain. The lips and gums are less commonly affected. Leukoplakic areas can occasionally occur on the dorsal aspect of the tongue. Oral lichen planus may persist for a long time if not treated with steroids. The skin lesions consist of itchy, flat-topped violaceous papules affecting the flexures of limbs. If there are severe oral lesions and extensive involvement of skin, systemic steroids may be indicated. Most of the lesions are suppressed with topical steroid applications.

Mucous membrane pemphigoid

This develops commonly in the mucosa of the eyes or mouth and may persist for a long time. The blisters in the mouth rupture and produce painful ulcers. This condition is seen in elderly women and is rare. Diagnosis is made histologically and by immunofluorescence.

Oral candidosis

Monilial candida infection of the mouth is usually secondary to tetracycline therapy or an immunosuppressive regime of drugs. In infancy and childhood, it is seen as 'thrush' on the tongue or buccal mucosa. Persistent candidosis in adults may be a complication of endocrinopathy such as parathyroid disease. Treatment of candidosis is with topical nystatin mixture or amphotericin lozenges. Oral nystatin tablets may be required in persistent candidosis (p.104).

Eczema and dermatitis

Eczema and dermatitis are used synonymously for a group of disorders which produce an acute, subacute or chronic inflammatory reaction of skin. They appear as erythema, oedema and vesicles producing itchy weeping and crusting lesions. Scratching of the lesions produces excoriation and lichenification.

Atopic eczema

A familial skin disorder characterized by the triad of asthma, eczema and hay fever. Those affected show an increased tendency to hypersensitivity to protein and other substances.

In infantile eczema, the flexures of groins, elbows, knees and face are usually affected.

In the adult type, the eczema produces lichenified patches on the flexures of limbs with excoriations and secondary infection.

Treatment consists of emollients such as emulsifying ointment BP, topical steroids for suppression of active dermatitis and control of secondary infection.

Contact eczema

The dermatitis may be due to primary irritant reactions or secondary sensitization to allergenic substances.

A primary irritant is a substance which produces an acute inflammation of the skin at first contact for a sufficient length of time. It is self-limiting and clears rapidly once the irritant is removed. Allergic contact sensitivity requires repeated exposures to the sensitizer such as nickel, perfumes, rubber and dyes.

Identification of the cause requires detailed history, occupation, hobbies and other factors.

Diagnosis is confirmed by patch testing to the relevant contactant. The patch test is based on the assumption that if a substance causes dermatitis, it should reproduce an inflammatory reaction when applied to an unaffected area of skin.

Topical applications of antibiotics like neomycin, chloramphenicol or antihistamine creams or local anaesthetics of the procaine series are potential sensitizers, and should therefore be avoided.

Drug eruptions

The skin eruptions induced by systemic drugs are the result of an immunological reaction to the medications. Occasionally a pharmacological adverse reaction may be a factor. The types of immunological reactions caused by drugs can be classified as:

Type I   Anaphylactic reactions.
Type II   Cytotoxic reactions.
Type III   Immune complex-mediated reactions.
Type IV   Cell-mediated or delayed hypersensitivity.

The drug reactions present as widespread blotchy erythematous lesions symmetrical in distribution, or they may produce an urticarial rash. The rash usually develops suddenly. Fever and lymphadeno-pathy may accompany the rash. The pattern and type of rash is outlined as:

Erythema multiforme—sulphonamides, penicillins
Urticarial lesions—aspirin, penicillins
Blistering lesions—barbiturates, sedatives
Lichenoid eruptions—anti-malarials, methyldopa
Acneiform papules—anti-tuberculous drugs, anti-epileptics
Photoallergic rash—chlorpromazine, sulphonylureas
Fixed drug eruptions—phenacetin, phenylbutazones
Purpura—thiazides, indomethacin
Exfoliative dermatitis—gold salts, phenylbutazone

Cross-sensitization may occur if the patient is sensitized to a particular drug and if exposed to a chemically related but different drug.

There is no specific skin test for a drug reaction. The 'challenge test' can be used occasionally in mild drug eruptions but may be hazardous in precipitating an anaphylactic reaction, e.g. penicillin. Patch tests are useful only in epidermal reactions. Prick tests are risky and unreliable. Desensitization is an unrewarding procedure and the patient should be warned of the risk involved.

Adverse skin reaction due to topical applications

The topical antihistamine creams may cause acute eczematous reactions on an already inflamed skin such as caused by insect bites. Repeated use of the creams on the exposed areas of skin may precipitate an acute photosensitive dermatitis. They are potent skin sensitizers and may react violently on challenge to either systemic or topical use of the offending antihistamine. In fact the topical anti-histamines have no therapeutic value in dermatological use.

Topical anaesthetic creams of the procaine series are potential sensitizers. Antibiotics like neomycin and chloramphenicol are well-known sensitizers and should be used with caution.

Long-term use of fluorinated steroid creams produces atrophy of the epidermis, with thinning of the skin, fragility, spontaneous bruising, striae, persistent telangiectasia with loss of dermal collagen. The adverse effects are reversible on withdrawal after a prolonged interval, except for the telangiectasia and striae. The misuse of topical steroids may produce an entity known as 'tinea incognito' which is an atypical fungal superinfection of the treated area. Scabetic infestation could be masked by misuse of topical steroid creams.

Cutaneous infections and infestation

Normal skin is colonized by organisms which are commensals such as Gram-positive cocci, diphtheroids, candida and acne bacilli. They harbour in sebaceous glands, hair follicles and crypts. The potential pathogens become active and cause infection when there is fissuring or active dermatitis.

Impetigo

A superficial infection caused by staphylococci or streptococci. It is common in childhood and affects the skin or face around the mouth and nose. The lesions develop as thin-walled blisters which rupture easily and form golden yellow-coloured crusts. They appear rapidly on an active dermatitis or atopic eczema.

Treatment consists of removal of crust with saline soaks or antiseptics and a topical antibiotic like fucidin or tetracycline may be sufficient. Bacteriological confirmation of the cause of the lesion is useful for selecting an appropriate antibiotic.

Erysipelas

A streptococcal infection characterized by sharply demarcated erythematous lesions usually on the face. The infection follows an abrasion or injury to skin. The patient may be ill with fever or rigor. Penicillin is the drug of choice.

Cellulitis

A streptococcal infection through a portal of entry in the skin. The legs are usually affected. The attack is acute in onset, with high fever and rigors and also regional lymphadenopathy. Recurrent episodes cause lymphoedema. Penicillin controls the infection rapidly.

Folliculitis

A chronic staphylococcal infection affecting the hair follicles, commonly in the beard area. Chronic nasal infection or foci of sepsis such as otitis externa or in the throat may be the precipitating cause. The lesions are follicular pustules with surrounding redness. Topical sodium fusidate or chlortetracycline and eradication of focal sepsis should clear the lesions.

Scabies

This is a contagious disease caused by an acarus mite (sarcoptes scabiei). This is characterized by burrows, follicular papules with severe pruritus worse at night. One or all members of the family may be affected. Treatment with gamma benzene hexachloride or benzyl benzoate for two nights followed by a scrub bath should clear the infestation. All the affected members should be treated simultaneously.

Pediculosis
This infestation is caused by three types of lice. They are the scalp, body and pubic lice. The condition is mostly evident in young girls and women under unhygienic environment especially due to sexual contact. The diagnosis is confirmed by the demonstration of translucent nits attached to hair roots and moving lice in the hairy areas. Treatment is aimed at eradication of the nits and delousing with dicophane lotions or gamma benzene hexachloride lotion. The beddings and clothes require thorough washing and laundering.

Fungus infections
Fungal infection is characterized by itchy scaly lesions which spread peripherally affecting the groins, axillae, soles, scalp and the nails. There are three common generic types of fungi, namely trichophyton, microsporum and epidermophyton. The nail affection produces brittle dystrophic lesions which are usually asymptomatic. Diagnosis is confirmed by direct microscopy with potassium hydroxide for hyphae. Wood's light examination of the scalp shows brilliant fluorescence. The fungi are cultured in Sabouraud's medium. Anti-fungal antibiotics such as griseofulvin and recently ketoconazole are used systemically with good results. Topical miconazole and econazole lotions and creams are effective in superficial infections.

Viral infections
The common warts are benign skin tumours, usually self-limiting, multiple raised lesions found on the back of the hands. They are caused by human papilloma virus. Spread of infection occurs among school children and in swimming pools. Most of the lesions clear spontaneously within a period of two years. The resistant warts require treatment with liquid nitrogen spray, or topical wart paints containing gluteraldehyde or salicyclic/lactic acid lotions are usually effective.

Molluscum contagiosum
This is caused by a pox virus, commonly seen in children. The lesions occur on the face, neck or on the trunk. They are reddish small

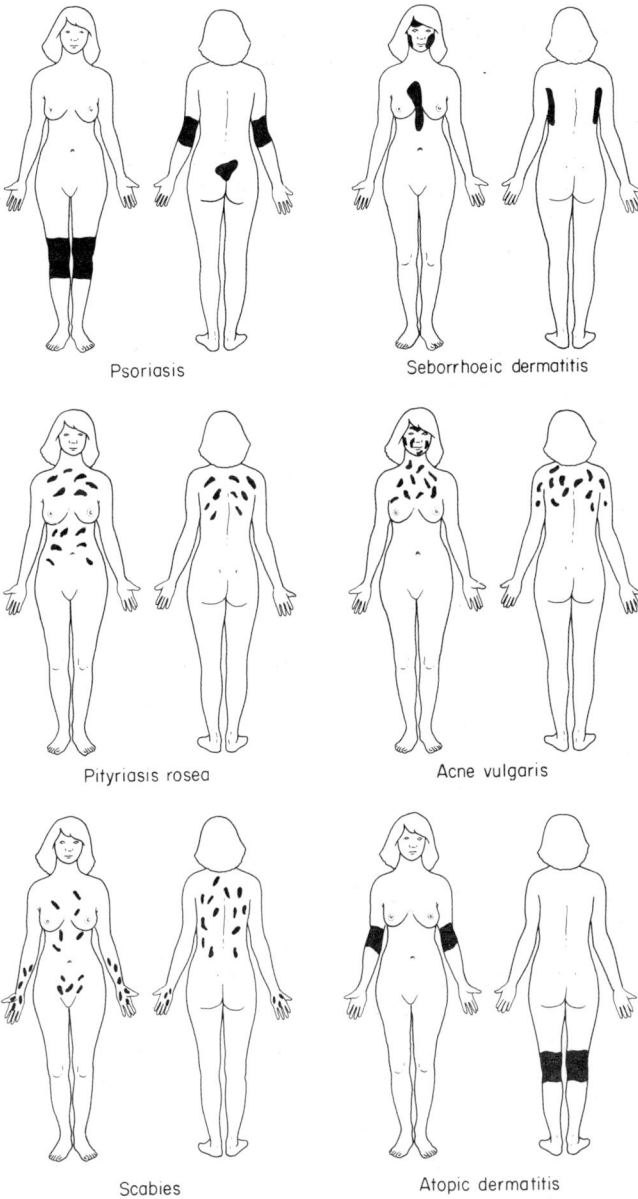

Fig. 12 Distribution of common skin lesions.

papules with a characteristic central punctum. Multiple satellite lesions develop on the same skin, and may rupture. Treatment with liquid nitrogen spray or carbon dioxide in acetone slush is effective.

Orf
This pox virus infection occurs as a solitary, rapidly growing nodule through contact with an infected sheep. Common among agricultural workers. Spontaneous recovery takes place after a period of one or two weeks after reaching a necrotic centre or nodule. Topical treatment with tetracycline ointment prevents secondary infection and scarring.

Erythemato-squamous disorders
This group of skin disorders is characterized by scaling and redness. The common disorders are psoriasis, seborrhoeic dermatitis, pityriasis rosea and exfoliative dermatitis.

Psoriasis
This is a chronic recurring inflammatory disease, characterized by well-defined papules or large plaques of varying sizes and shapes, affecting the extensor aspect of elbows, knees, scalp, trunk and abdomen. The sexes are equally affected and the incidence is about 2–3% of the population. Any age may be affected. The familial incidence is about 25–30%. The precipitating factors of this disease are acute infections, injury and emotional upsets.

The lesions develop as small silvery scales and papules which on scratching flake easily producing punctate bleeding bases. The papules gradually enlarge producing plaques of various sizes. Most of the lesions are not itchy but at times can be. The nails are often involved with pitting, thickening and brownish yellow staining at the edges. Arthritis of the sacro-iliac joints and terminal interphalangeal joints is common. Pustular psoriasis of the palms and soles is a variant of psoriasis which is usually chronic and difficult to treat.

Treatment is aimed at descaling of the lesions with various tar and dithranol preparations. Ultraviolet light is used in combination with tar or systemic psoralen compounds (PUVA). The steroids used topically have a very limited place in the long-term management. Cytotoxic drugs such as methotrexate and hydroxyurea are used in severe types of psoriasis.

Seborrhoeic dermatitis
This is an acute or chronic scaly disorder of the hairy areas of the scalp, presterum, axillae and groins. The eyebrows and face are often involved with greasy scaling. The condition may recur in the scalp and may require prolonged therapy with sulphur/salicylic ointment.

Pityriasis rosea
This is a mild inflammatory disorder characterized by superficial circinate scaly lesions on the trunk. The condition starts as a symptomless, solitary macular 'herald patch' on the trunk and after a week or two, symmetrical maculopapular lesions develop on the trunk or arms. The lesions resolve spontaneously within eight to ten weeks. The aetiology is unknown.

Exfoliative dermatitis
This is seen as a generalized erythroderma. It is usually a complication of a pre-existing skin disease such as eczema, psoriasis or skin lymphoma or drug eruption. The skin disease is accompanied by constitutional symptoms. Treatment is bed-rest, maintenance of fluid balance and treating the underlying disease. Systemic steroids are used to control the symptoms. Prognosis depends on the primary skin disease.

Bullous diseases
The bullous diseases of the skin are classified as follows:

Table 12 Bullous skin diseases.

Intra-epidermal blisters	Sub-epidermal blisters
Eczema/dermatitis	Erythema multiforme
Infection	Dermatitis herpetiformis
Trauma	Bullous pemphigoid
Pemphigus vulgaris	Porphyria

The intra-epidermal blisters rupture very easily and the subepidermal blisters are tense and intact.

Eczema/dermatitis
This develops as small multiloculated vesiculo-papules which coalesce to produce an eczematous reaction.

Infections
In bullous impetigo and herpetic lesions, the blisters rupture and form crusts.

Pemphigus vulgaris
An uncommon blistering disorder of unknown aetiology, which affects middle-aged persons. It develops slowly with widespread flaccid bullae affecting the skin and erosions of buccal mucosa, eyes, genitalia and anus. It is diagnosed by biopsy of a bulla which shows an intra-epidermal blister with acantholytic cells. Immunofluorescence studies confirm the diagnosis. High-dose steroid therapy controls the disease.

Dermatitis herpetiformis
Develops as itchy papules and small groups of blisters, usually on the extensor aspects of the elbows, shoulders, sacrum and knees. The disease is associated with intestinal lesions, as in coeliac disease. Flattening of the jejunal mucosa and gluten enteropathy can be demonstrated. Diagnosis is by biopsy of the blister which shows a subepidermal blister and is confirmed by immunofluorescence. Treatment is specific with dapsone and gluten-free diet.

Bullous pemphigoid
Usually affects the older age group. This condition may be associated with other auto-immune diseases. The blisters develop on itchy skin and are usually large, tense and filled with clear or blood-stained serum. Diagnosis is confirmed by histology showing a subepidermal bulla and immunofluorescence at the basement membrane. Treatment is with steroids.

Porphyria
The blisters in cutaneous porphyria appear on the sun-exposed areas of face, back of hands and scalp. The blisters may appear after trauma. Hepatotoxic chemicals or alcohol may produce skin lesions. Diagnosis is by determination of porphyrins in faeces, urine and blood. Wood's light examination for red fluorescence is confirmatory. Drugs like sulphonamides, barbiturates and griseofulvin are contraindicated.

24   ENT disorders

Nasal haemorrhage (epistaxis)
Bleeding from the nose is a common and occasionally serious condition. The bleeding usually comes from Little's area on the anterior part of the septum which has a rich, anastomotic blood supply, receiving branches from the anterior ethmoidal, greater palatine, sphenopalatine and superior labial arteries. Less commonly, bleeding comes from the lateral wall of the nose which receives most of its blood supply from the sphenopalatine and ethmoidal arteries. The upper part of the nasal septum is supplied by the posterior ethmoidal artery. Bleeding from the nose may be caused by local lesions or it may be associated with general conditions:

Local
1. *Spontaneous.* Bleeding, which tends to recur, comes from Little's area ar ' is common in healthy young people.
2. *Trauma.*
3. *Atrophic rhinitis (rhinitis medicamentosa).* Caused by excessive use of nasal decongestants.
4. *Hereditary haemorrhagic telangiectasia (Osler–Weber–Rendu disease).* In this rare familial disorder, telangiectases occur in the skin and mucous membranes of the nose, mouth and tongue, and of the gastrointestinal, respiratory and renal tracts. Bleeding from the nose and gut usually occurs only in adult life and may lead to severe iron deficiency anaemia.
5. *Tumours of the nose and sinuses.* Especially in middle age.

General

Hypertension. Severe, prolonged, recurrent epistaxis from the posterior part of the nose may occur in middle-aged and elderly hypertensive patients, but it is uncertain how much this is caused by the raised blood pressure rather than simply by diseased or aged blood vessels.

General bleeding disorders. These include the leukaemias, purpuric state, haemophilia, von Willebrand's disease, scurvy and vitamin K deficiency.

Anticoagulant drugs.

Liver disease. Epistaxis is uncommon, but is especially likely to occur when liver disease is associated with jaundice.

Renal failure. Especially when associated with hypertension.

Treatment
1. Simple pressure is usually sufficient to stop bleeding from Little's area.
2. When simple pressure fails to stop bleeding, anterior nasal packing with half-inch ribbon gauze moistened with equal parts of 4% lignocaine and 1:1000 adrenaline (epinephrine) solution should be used for 10–15 min to anaesthetize the nose and give some vaso-constriction, the anaesthetic pack removed, and a Vaseline ribbon gauze pack substituted and left in position for 24 hours.
   (*Do not leave lignocaine and adrenaline packs in for 24 hours.*)
3. Posterior and nasal packing may be required, particularly in hyper-tensive patients.
4. Cautery: after anaesthetizing locally, the bleeding point is touched with trichloracetic acid, a chromic acid bead, or a silver nitrate applicator. Galvano (electric) cautery may be used in adults.
5. Oestrogens may be used to cause hypertrophy of the nasal mucous membrane, especially in patients with hereditary telangiectasia.
6. Treatment of the underlying medical condition.
7. Correction of anaemia with oral iron therapy or blood transfusion according to its severity.

Note. Epistaxis is occasionally a sign of a serious underlying disorder.

Maxillary sinusitis
Each maxillary sinus (antrum) is a pyramidal-shaped cavity lined with ciliated columnar epithelium containing numerous cells which secrete mucus. Normally the mucus is continually swept by the cilia towards an opening (the ostium) which lies in the upper part of the median wall and leads into the middle nasal meatus. The bucco-alveolar sulcus is

anterior to the antrum and the lateral part of the hard palate and the roots of the second premolar and first two molar teeth lie inferiorly.

Inflammation of the lining of the antrum or any of the other paranasal air sinuses is called sinusitis. The disorder produces definite signs and symptoms but despite this it is overdiagnosed. Maxillary sinusitis is the commonest form of the disorder and is the only variety which has direct relevance to dental practice.

Types

(1) *Suppurative*
    Acute,
    Subacute,
    Chronic.
(2) Allergic

Acute suppurative maxillary sinusitis is commonly caused by:
1. The common cold or influenza.
2. 10% are secondary to extraction or apical infection of the premolar or molar teeth, particularly first/second molars.
3. The most common responsible organisms (based on non-contaminated cultures obtained by direct antral puncture) are:
(i)   *Haemophilus influenzae.*
(ii)   *Streptococcus pneumoniae* (pneumococcus).
(iii) Bacteria not usually found in the nose and mouth, e.g. *E.coli* and anaerobic streptococci, the latter causing foul-smelling pus.
(iv) Adenovirus.

Note. Other causes include fractures of the alveolus, swimming, diving (both scuba and sky) and barotrauma.

Its clinical features include a gradual onset of stuffy nose and a feeling of pressure over the sinus. Mild general malaise and headache are common, but significant pyrexia and leucocytosis are unusual. Severe pain and tenderness sharply localized over the cheek and several or all of the upper teeth appear within 48–72 hours. The adjacent nasal mucosa is hyperaemic and oedematous and produces a purulent discharge. Acute maxillary sinusitis causes symptoms which may be confused with a few other disorders:
a. Pain of dental origin (dental abscess).
b. Trigeminal neuralgia–involving the second division of the 5th cranial nerve (pp.176 & 186).
c. Neoplasm of the sinus (p.277).
d. Erysipelas. (p.261).

To investigate, use:
1. Transillumination: the antrum fails to transmit light.
2. X-ray: clouding of the sinus and sometimes a fluid level may be seen.
3. Proof puncture, washout and culture.

Notes. The clinical characteristics of sinusitis do not clearly differentiate a normal from an abnormal sinus. Typical symptoms may be associated with normal antral puncture. Typical purulent sinusitis diagnosed by antral puncture may be entirely asymptomatic.

Principles of treatment are:
1. The restoration of patency of nasal airways and the ostium of the sinus (to promote reventilation and drainage of the antrum): nasal decongestants, e.g. 1–2% ephedrine in normal saline.
2. Analgesics.
3. Antibiotics: may be used if pain persists together with fever and a significant leucocytosis. The symptoms usually settle spontaneously after 3– 4 days. When antibiotics are used the drug of choice should be amoxycillin unless otherwise indicated by the culture of sinus fluid obtained on proof puncture.
4. Puncture of the thin medial (non-diploetic) bony wall of the antrum and washout are necessary only when medical treatment is ineffective as a result of complete occlusion of the ostium by mucosal oedema and the purulent discharge. The antrum then fills with pus under pressure (antral empyema), pain becomes unbearable and the infection may spread.

Notes. Any tooth or dental root retained within the sinus should be removed as soon as possible. Maxillary sinusitis secondary to an oroantral fistula is considered on p.276. Secondary intracranial infection as a result of venous spread via the pterygoid plexus is rare in antral infections. In infants, acute infection of the dental sac following injury occasionally leads to osteomyelitis of the alveolus and hard palate and to antral empyema.

Prognosis
90% are cured by conservative treatment; the others persist in a subacute form.

Subacute suppurative sinusitis has only one constant clinical feature, this being a persistent purulent nasal discharge. Tenderness is absent but there may be vague, intermittent discomfort over the sinus. Allergy is sometimes an important contributory factor.

Investigation
1. The antrum fails to transilluminate.
2. X-rays determine which other sinuses are involved.
3. Culture of the sinus washings obtained on proof puncture is helpful; culture of the nasal discharge gives unreliable information.

Principles of treatment are:
1. *Antral irrigation*: needle through medial wall of sinus (antral puncture). Normal mucosal ciliary activity often returns within a few hours of the procedure and further clearance of the purulent sinus contents occurs spontaneously.
2. *Antibiotic-containing solutions* are sometimes used for the irrigation but their use is not essential.

Notes. Satisfactory treatment prevents the disorder from becoming chronic. When the above treatment fails, the antrum should be permanently drained by making an antral 'window' through the lateral wall of the nose under the inferior turbinate (p.272).

Chronic suppurative sinusitis is characterized by irreversible inflammatory changes in the antral mucosa. These result from neglected subacute sinusitis or from repeated acute attacks. The clininal features are the same as those of the subacute form but manifestations of allergy are more common. Pain is absent: persistent pain over the sinus should indicate an impending complication or an unsuspected neoplasm (p.277). The investigations used are the same as those for subacute sinusitis.

Notes. The information obtained from transillumination, X-ray films and irrigation and culture, is not always in accord. However, in patients with acute symptoms an antrum opaque to transillumination strongly suggests sinus infection, whereas in patients with prolonged symptoms it suggests a sinus abnormality with or without infection. Normal transillumination is a not very helpful finding and mucosal thickening apparent on the X-ray, unless marked, is an unreliable indicator of sinus infection. Antral puncture, followed by culture and determination of the leucocyte content of the sinus aspirate, is the most reliable diagnostic procedure.

To treat chronic sinusitis it is necessary to remove all of the diseased soft tissue and to ensure adequate post-operative drainage. These objectives are achieved by means of a radical operation such as the *Caldwell–Luc* procedure.

Note on the Caldwell–Luc operation. A temporary 'window' is made into the antrum through the canine fossa to facilitate removal of all of the diseased mucosa and periosteum; the bony antro-nasal wall below the attachment of the inferior nasal turbinate is then removed to ensure permanent good drainage from the bottom of the sinus, the adjacent nasal mucosa and periosteum being preserved as a flap which is turned in to the antral floor. The exposed antral bone becomes recovered by nasal mucosa.

Allergic sinusitis. This is an integral part of the allergic syndrome which is characterized by nasal stuffiness, itching and burning, frequent sneezing and a thin nasal discharge. Mucosal polyps are common both in the sinuses and in the nose. Antihistamines are the mainstay of treatment.

Note. Superimposed suppurative and allergic sinusitis is termed *hyperplastic* because of the resultant severe tissue oedema, mucosal polyps and chronic thickening of the mucosa and submucosa that block the ostium. Antihistamines and excision of the diseased soft tissue are helpful but the nasal symptoms usually persist.

Oro-antral fistula

An oro-antral fistula is a communication between the maxillary sinus (antrum) and the oral cavity. Such fistulae are probably more common than is generally realized. Most are caused by dental trauma, especially extractions, and many of these escape diagnosis and heal spontaneously without complications.

Other causes include:
1. Penetrating wounds to the upper jaw, e.g. gun shot wounds.
2. Fractures of the maxilla.
3. Maxillary sinus operations: when the temporary oral incision fails to heal (p.272).
4. Neoplastic erosion of the maxilla (usually from within the antrum) (p.277).
5. Excision of a maxillary tumour.

Fistulae of dental origin

Predisposing causes

Abnormally thin or deficient bony antral floor. Extraction of a molar or premolar tooth then invariably tears the antral mucosa and produces a fistula.

Abnormal pneumatization of the maxillary tuberosity. A very large fistula may be caused during the extraction of a posterior molar tooth as the entire weakened tuberosity may remain attached to the tooth.

Localized sclerosis of bone. The brittle bone may be ankylosed to the teeth so that a post-extraction fistula is inevitable.

Hypercementosis. Abnormal cementum deposits are laid down around the roots of the teeth which become bulbous as a result. Associated bone sclerosis is common and ankylosis extreme. Surgical removal of bone is essential to permit safe delivery of the teeth, but fistula formation may still occur.

Tortuous dental roots. May have claw-like grip on surrounding bone which separates with fistula formation during extraction—especially common during extraction of trifurcated first molar tooth.

Softening and erosion of alveolar bone. May be associated with apical abscess or antral carcinoma. The post-extraction fistula that results may be the first indication of the tumour.

Excessive force. Large fragments of normal bone may occasionally be torn out during an extraction. The risk is proportional to the force used.

Search for retained root fragments. An elevator or other instrument inserted to remove a broken palatal root of a first molar tooth displaced between the alveolus and the antral mucosa can easily perforate the antral lining and thus create a fistula.

Clincal features and diagnosis
1. Frequently immediately obvious after dental extraction.
2. Patients may complain later of:
   (i) Pain over the maxillary sinus (common).
   (ii) Air or fluids being sucked through the fistula into the nose.
   (iii) Poor retention of denture fitted after the extraction.
   (iv) Foul, purulent discharge from mouth or nose.
3. If diagnosis in doubt, one can:
   (i) Pass probe through tooth socket into antrum.
   (ii) Inject contrast medium through the fistula, then X-ray.
   (iii) Inject fluid through the fistula to demonstrate a communication between the antrum and the nose.

Notes. These investigations help to exclude the diagnosis of *pseudofistula* (an alveolar opening ending blindly in a dental cyst). Radiological examination is mandatory is all cases of suspected or clinically obvious oro-antral fistula. The X-ray films may show:
(i) Retained tooth roots.
(ii) Foreign bodies.
(iii) Evidence consistent with antral infection (p.269).

Management

Natural healing. May take place by primary or secondary intention (p.21).
1. *Primary healing*: most fistulae will heal spontaneously provided a blood clot fills the defect and is not disturbed. The clot is replaced quickly by granulation tissue and then fibrous tissue; finally, mucosal integrity is restored both in the antrum and in the mouth.
2. *Secondary healing*: primary healing may be interrupted and the exposed tissues become raw, swollen and granular. Spontaneous secondary healing may still occur once the exposed tissues become adherent over the defect, but only if the fistula is small. There are several causes of interrupted primary healing:
   (i) Defect is so large that the blood clot is unstable or insufficient to plug the gap.
   (ii) Clot disintegration caused by early infection.
   (iii) Dislodgement of the clot by vigorous probing, syringing or excessive mouth washes.
   (iv) Malignant disease—usually of the antrum (p.277).

Note. Very large fistulae cannot close either by primary or by secondary intention. The mucosa cannot bridge the gap either in the mouth or in the antrum. Instead it grows down the fistulous tract from each end and completely epithelializes it, spontaneous closure is thus rendered impossible (p.22).

Surgical closure. The two most important factors that determine the type of treatment given are the delay before the patient is seen and whether or not the antrum is infected. The surgical management can conveniently be considered for three categories of fistulae:
1. *Recent*: less than 24 hours old.
2. *Intermediate*: between 1 and 14 days old.
3. *Late*: well established.

1. *Recent fistulae.* The antrum is usually not infected in the first 24 hours and the sooner the fistula is closed the less likely is it to become so. Primary operative repair is therefore preferable to conservative treatment, especially as it makes successful fistula repair more certain:
   (a) *Small fistulae*: can be closed in the dental surgery.
   (b) *Large fistulae*: should be closed in hospital using an advancement or rotation flap.

Notes. Mobilization of the gum round the socket, relief incisions and trimming of the bony socket edges may be required to avoid suture-line tension. Trimming must leave sufficient bone to support a denture. Nose-blowing must be avoided until the fistula has healed. Systemic antibiotics must be given for at least 5 days.

2. *Intermediate fistulae.* When antibiotics have not been given, low-grade infection is invariable in fistulae first seen between 1 and 14 days after their creation. The traumatized tissues are therefore granular and friable and this precludes sound surgical repair. Fortunately, most will close spontaneously within four weeks provided:
   (a) The clot filling the fistula is not disturbed—probing and irrigation are therefore forbidden and sucking and blowing through the fistula must be avoided. The fistula should be protected by a prosthesis.
   (b) A systemic antibiotic, e.g. penicillin, is given.

Notes. Four months may be required for the spontaneous healing of very large intermediate fistulae. Spontaneous closure after 4 months is unlikely.

3. *Late fistulae*. Four factors predispose to fistulae becoming well established:
   (a) Epithelialization of the tract,
   (b) Pre-existing chronic maxillary sinusitis,
   (c) Osteomyelitis of the alveolar process of the maxilla,
   (d) An unusually large bony defect.

After the cure of an antral infection, gentle curettage of the tract (i.e. sufficient to cause bleeding) or the application of sclerosing solution may denude the tract of its epithelium and so restimulate the healing of late small fistulae, but operative repair is usually required. It is preferable to use a two-layer closure for the repair, the first layer consisting of infolded buccal epithelium from the margins of the fistula and the outer part of the tract, the second consisting of a buccal or palatal mucoperiosteal flap. Sometimes, especially if the fistula is very large, it is necessary to excise completely the outer part of the epithelialized tract and close the fistula with the mucoperiosteal flap alone. Protective splinting is of doubtful value.

Factors complicating fistula repair
1. *Adjacent teeth*
   (a) *Teeth with exposed roots*: prior removal may facilitate survival of the soft tissue flap.
   (b) *Solitary tooth*: best to retain as a denture support, especially if at distal end of an edentulous region of the maxilla and other sound teeth are present in the upper jaw.
   (c) *Teeth requiring extraction*: best removed several weeks before the fistula repair to allow sockets to epithelialize.
2. *Retained dental roots*
   X-rays in at least two head positions are necessary to demonstrate their exact positions. Their early removal avoids later infection.
   (i) In substance of alveolus: dental surgeon should remove.
   (ii) Free within antral cavity: ENT surgeon should remove via a canine fossa (Caldwell–Luc) approach. If associated with antral infection, retained roots are best removed during a procedure designed to eradicate it (p.272).
3. *Maxillary sinus infection*
   Common, especially in presence of dental or gingival disease. Repeated probing, socket lavage and lack of fistula protection at meal times increase the risk. When the infection is severe the antrum

may fill with pus. Acute infections respond favourably to systemic antibiotics but severe infections also need regular antral lavage (usually through the fistula) and the local instillation of an appropriate antibiotic preparation for their control. Chronic infections usually predate the fistulae and require combined radical antrostomy (Caldwell–Luc type, p.272) and fistula repair for their cure.

Note on the prostheses in oro-antral fistulae. Rarely a well-made permanent appliance is used to close the fistula, as, for example, in patients who refuse surgical repair, the very old or medically unfit, or when repeated surgical attempts at closure have failed. Temporary prostheses have limited application in conservative treatment.

Antral carcinoma
The earliest feature of antral carcinoma is the appearance of blood in a chronic nasal discharge. This may be accompanied by swelling of the cheek and swelling or ulceration of the bucco-alveolar sulcus, perhaps with the formation of an oro-antral fistula. Proptosis (bulging forward of the eye), diplopia (double vision), and watering of the eye may occur because of orbital spread. Facial pain may occur in the distribution of the maxillary division of the trigeminal nerve, but the pain is occasionally referred to areas supplied by the ophthalmic or mandibular divisions of the nerve. Lymphatic spread involves the submandibular and deep cervical lymph nodes. X-rays may show destruction of the bony antral walls and antral washings or a biopsy may reveal malignant cells.

Treatment
(a) Radiotherapy.
(b) Later, the hard palate on the affected side is removed, the subsequent fitting of a dental plate allowing regular inspection of the antrum and destruction of any local recurrence by means of diathermy.

Note. These measures achieve a 10–15% 5-year survival rate.

Disorders of the tonsils

Important indications for tonsillectomy
1. Recurrent attacks of acute tonsillitis, especially when they involve frequent absences from school or from work, or impair appetite.
2. Middle ear infection (adenoids must be removed as well).
3. Quinsy.
4. Persistent cervical lymph node enlargement after tonsillitis.
5. Progressive, unilateral tonsillar enlargement, as this may be caused by malignant disease.

Note. Other indications for tonsillectomy are conjectural and the operation is now less often performed.

Differential diagnosis of hoarseness
1. Chronic laryngitis: may result from misuse of voice, excessive use of alcohol or tobacco, or chronic sinusitis.
2. Leukoplakia of the larynx: malignant change may follow.
3. Benign or malignant laryngeal tumours.
4. Vocal cord paresis.
5. Myxoedema.
6. Laryngeal oedema from any cause.
7. Pharyngeal tumours.
8. Laryngeal tuberculosis: associated with pulmonary tuberculosis.
9. Syphilitic laryngitis: gummatous infiltration: rare.

Treatment. That of the underlying disorder.

The causes of earache
1. Furunculosis of the external ear.
2. Acute middle ear infection (otitis media).
3. Referred earache (*see* below).
4. Acute mastoiditis.
5. Malignant disease of the external or middle ear.

Note on referred earache. Pain may be referred to the ear from lesions within the distribution of the following nerves: Auriculotemporal branch of the trigeminal, e.g. impacted lower molar teeth, disturbances of the temporo-mandibular joint, sphenoidal sinusitis; sensory branch of the facial e.g. geniculate herpes; tympanic branch of the glossopharyngeal and auricular branch of the vagus, e.g. glossopharyngeal neuralgia, tonsillar disorders or malignant disease of the posterior third of the tongue, vallecula, lateral pharyngeal wall, hypopharynx or larynx; great auricular (2nd and 3rd cervical nerve fibres), e.g. cervical spondylosis.

Acute middle ear infection (acute otitis media)
Acute throbbing pain in the ear is associated with pyrexia and malaise. The infection occurs in association with a streptococcal upper respiratory tract infection and blockage of the eustachian tube.

Treatment. Penicillin.

Complications
1. Perforation of the ear drum,
2. Acute mastoiditis,
3. Meningitis,
4. Extradural, subdural, temporal lobe or cerebellar abscess,
5. Facial paralysis caused by involvement of the VIIth nerve in its course through the middle ear,
6. Labyrinthitis,
7. Lateral sinus thrombosis.

Tinnitus
This is a sensation of buzzing, hissing or ringing noises in the ear. The causes of the disorder include:
1. Wax in the external auditory canal impacted against the drum.
2. Chronic middle ear disease.
3. Otosclerosis: this is characterized by new bone formation around the footplate of the stapes with consequent ankylosis. Deafness is also a prominent feature.
4. Ménière's disease (p.281).
5. Sensori-neural deafness from any cause, e.g. presbycusis (senile deafness), noise-induced, e.g. air-drills.
6. Drugs, especially toxic doses of salicylates or aminoglycoside antibiotics, e.g. streptomycin, neomycin.

Note. Noise-induced deafness in boiler makers and drop forge workers has long been recognized. Modern causes include 'pop-group' deafness, discos and air-drills.

Vertigo
This is a sensation of rotation in space, either vertically or horizontally, and may involve the patient or his surroundings. It is important to distinguish true vertigo from other similar forms of sensory disturbance such as a feeling of being about to faint or to fall to one or other side. True vertigo has a number of important causes:

1. Labyrinthine disorders:
   (a) Ménière's disease (p.281).
   (b) Vestibular neuronitis (epidemic vertigo): this disorder is thought to be caused by a virus infection and the illness is usually self-limiting.
   (c) Benign positional vertigo: common in the elderly.
2. VIIIth nerve damage induced by drugs, e.g. streptomycin.
3. Disease of the central nervous system:
   (a) Multiple sclerosis (p.172).
   (b) Brain-stem vascular disorders (p.178).
   (c) Acoustic neurinoma.
4. Geniculate herpes (Ramsay Hunt syndrome).

Common causes of deafness
1. Wax in the external ear,
2. Acute or chronic middle ear infection,
3. Secretory or catarrhal middle ear disease following acute upper respiratory tract infections,
4. Damage caused by abrupt changes in atmospheric pressure (barotrauma),
5. Otosclerosis,
6. Presbycusis,
7. Acute systemic infections, e.g. measles,
8. Tympanic membrane injuries,
9. Congenital, e.g. rubella, syphilis,
10. Head injuries, e.g., skull fractures causing damage to the VIIIth nerve,
11. Ménière's disease (*see* p.281),
12. Drugs: streptomycin, neomycin, salicylates, quinine, and many others.

Ménière's disease

This disorder is characterized by intermittent vertigo, vomiting and deafness and is thought to be caused by distension of the membranous labyrinth with fluid.

Treatment. Antiemetic drugs, e.g. prochlorperazine (Stemetil).

Tracheostomy

This surgical procedure consists of removing a small part of the anterior surface of the trachea. The effect of this operation is to:
1. Facilitate the clearance of secretions from the trachea and main bronchi.
2. Reduce the physiological airways dead space.
3. Maintain an adequate airway over long periods, especially in the unconscious patient.
4. Permit mechanical ventilation.
5. Bypass upper airway (usually laryngeal) obstruction.

Note. Endotracheal tubes inserted via the pharyngeal route fulfil all the above requirements, but owing to the risk of damage from pressure on both the larynx and the trachea, such tubes should not be left in place for longer than about 7 days. If further intubation is required, tracheostomy is essential.

Indications for tracheostomy
1. *Laryngeal obstruction*
   (a) Oedema caused by allergy, infections such as laryngo-tracheo-bronchitis or diphtheria, or corrosive poisons, e.g., lysol.
   (b) Foreign bodies.
   (c) Trauma causing a laryngeal haematoma.

Note. The above constitute emergency indications for tracheostomy which is required to save life.

The features of acute laryngeal oedema with impending obstruction are:
1. Stridor: a harsh, crowing noise on inspiration.
2. Features of hypoxia: anxiety, restlessness, pallor, sweating and a fast pulse.
3. *Cyanosis complicating acute laryngeal obstruction is an indication for immediate intervention.*

Note. In children, indrawing of the suprasternal, intercostal and epigastric muscles is an additional sign of laryngeal obstruction.

2. *Failure to clear secretions from the trachea and bronchi*
   (a) Persistent, deep loss of consciousness, e.g. following head injury, poisoning or a stroke.
   (b) Bulbar palsy, e.g. poliomyelitis, polyneuritis or tetanus.
   (c) Pseudo-bulbar palsy, e.g. brain-stem ischaemia or a stroke.
   (d) Difficulty in coughing, e.g., chest injuries, neuromuscular disorders (e.g., poliomyelitis, myasthenia gravis) and severe respiratory disease (especially exacerbations of chronic bronchitis and postoperative pneumonia).

Notes. In group (d), tracheostomy has the beneficial effects of reducing the airways dead space and allowing artificial ventilation where required. Tracheostomy may be required to facilitate major operations in the oro-naso-pharyngeal region, or where trauma has produced major structural damage in this area.

Technique of the operation
1. In an emergency, a knife or scissors can be used to make a mid-line incision into the trachea just below the thyroid cartilage. Insertion of a tube through the wound will maintain an airway until skilled assistance is obtained.
2. Elective tracheostomy may be done under local or general anaesthesia. A transverse skin incision is made mid-way between the cricoid cartilage and the suprasternal notch. Vertical separation of the pre-tracheal muscles and the thyroid isthmus then precedes removal of a disc of tracheal tissue, including part of the 2nd to 4th tracheal rings. A polythene or silver tracheostomy tube is then inserted through the opening and its position secured with tapes.

Notes. Management of a tracheostomy includes the inspiration of humidified, warm air in order to keep the secretions loose and to prevent crusting and the formation of mucus plugs. The tracheostomy tube requires frequent cleaning. Heavy sedation must be avoided. When mechanical ventilation is required, a tracheostomy tube with an inflatable cuff is used. The purpose of the cuff is to prevent air escaping up through the larynx in the positive pressure phase of respiration. The pressure in the cuff must be released for five minutes in every hour to avoid pressure necrosis of the tracheal wall. Frequent suction of accumulated secretions in the trachea and main bronchi is also required.

25 Swellings of the neck and acute lesions of the mouth and throat

Neck swellings

Swellings in any region may be classified as: those structures which are normally present; those which are remnants of former embryological events; and those which arise outwith the region.

Swellings which are normally in the neck

In man, the Adam's apple, which is the thyroid cartilage in front of the larynx, is normally evident in the midline of the front of the neck. Many women have an easily visible thyroid gland just below this same site. The thyroid gland consists of two lobes joined by a narrow neck or isthmus. The whole gland may enlarge in response to increased demand, such as puberty or pregnancy, when the swelling seen is *physiological*. The whole gland may enlarge in association with overactivity (*thyrotoxicosis*) called *goitre* (p.137). These types of generalized swelling may be smooth or may be *multinodular*, which is a type of enlargement common in geographical areas where dietary iodine is deficient (p.166). Occasionally very large goitres can cause respiratory embarrassment. Another type of diffuse enlargement, but where the end result is a rather hard goitre, is an autoimmune condition known as *Hashimoto's disease*, which ends in *hypothyroidism* (p.139).

Sometimes, just part of the thyroid gland enlarges. This can be one lobe, or it can be a focus of tissue, anywhere within the gland, where it is known as a *solitary nodule*. These localized swellings can be either benign, an *adenoma,* or malignant, a *carcinoma*. There are four types of these malignancies:

1. *Papillary*: slow growing and relatively benign, tends to metastasize to lymph nodes in the neck which, in former years, when biopsied were considered to be *lateral aberrant thyroids*, commonest in young women.
2. *Follicular*: rather more malignant, although microscopically the appearances closely resemble normal thyroid tissue. When it

spreads, it does so to distant sites, particularly bone and lung. It occurs mostly in middle age.

3. *Anaplastic*, as the name implies, is usually very malignant, spreading chiefly locally. It occurs mainly in the elderly.
4. *Medullary* arises from *parafollicular* cells of the gland, responsible for secreting *thyrocalcitonin* and *prostaglandins*, excessive levels of which serve as detectable markers of this condition. It is associated with tumours of the adrenal gland (*phaeochromocytomas*) and cutaneous *neuromas*. Occasionally, a solitary thyroid nodule can be a *lymphoma*, which although radiosensitive has a poor prognosis, 75% of patients dying within 3 years of the diagnosis being made.

The lymph nodes of the neck are normally so small as to be invisible *and* impalpable. They enlarge in response to many different stimuli which can be classified as (1) *systemic* and (2) *local* and then subclassified into (i) *inflammatory* and (ii) *neoplastic* (Table 13).

Table 13 Causes of lymph node enlargement in the neck.

	Inflammatory	Neoplastic
Systemic	Glandular fever Sarcoidosis	Hodgkin's disease Lymphoma

	Tuberculosis	Lymphosarcoma
		Lymphatic leukaemia
		Secondary tumour, e.g.
		  breast, stomach,
		  lung

Local	Pharyngitis
	Tonsillitis
	Sepsis in face, neck or
	  mouth
		Carcinoma of pharynx
		Buccal cancer
		Cancer of lip
		Cancer of thyroid
		  (papillary)

	Quinsy Tinea capitis	Skin cancers Salivary gland tumours

The *salivary glands* at the junction of the face and neck are dealt with on p.113.

Swellings from embryological remnants
Since the thyroid has descended from the tongue, a midline remnant called a *thyroglossal cyst* can occur at any point from the back of the tongue to the upper trachea. Because of this origin, it moves with the tongue, but not with the larynx, in which respect it differs from the

thyroid gland itself (or a lump in that gland), which moves (with
the larynx) on swallowing.

Swellings in the lateral part of the neck can arise from the second
branchial cleft. So called *branchial cysts*, these are found in the upper
part of the neck just anterior to the upper third of the sternomastoid
muscle. They frequently present either as a discharging sinus or, as
their name implies, as a discrete cystic swelling, in young adult life.

Less discrete, softer swellings known as *cystic hygromas* sometimes
appear in infancy in the lateral part of the neck. These can be quite
difficult to excise completely.

Another neck swelling in infancy, the aetiology of which is
unknown, is a hard fibrous swelling which sometimes occurs in the
lower third of the sternomastoid, which left untreated may result in
shortening of the affected muscle and asymmetry of the developing
skull. This is called a sternomastoid tumour.

Swellings from outwith the neck
A number of tumours metastasize to skin. Adenocarcinoma of the
breast is the solid tumour most likely to give rise to nodules in
the skin of the neck, although gastric, pancreatic and renal tumours
spread this way, and some skin tumours, especially melanoma, have
a special propensity for causing deposits in skin at sites distant from
that of their origin.

Differential diagnosis of acute lesions of the mouth and throat

I *Infective causes:*

(a) *Bacterial infections*	*Streptococcus pyogenes, Staphylococcus aureas, Corynebacterium diphtheriae.*
(b) *Viral infections*	Epstein–Barr virus (glandular fever), herpes simplex, varicella zoster virus, Coxsackie viruses, adenovirus, other respiratory viruses.
(c) *Fungal infections*	*Candida albicans*, actinomycosis.
(d) *Spirochaetal infections*	Syphilis. Vincent's organisms.

II *Conditions of uncertain aetiology:*
  (a) Stevens–Johnson syndrome,
  (b) Behçet's syndrome.

III *Disorders of the blood:*
   (a) Agranulocytosis,
   (b) Aplastic anaemia,
   (c) Leukaemia.

IV *Neoplasms:*
Tumours of throat or mouth.

V *Trauma:*
Injuries to palate and pharynx. Foreign bodies.

Streptococcal and viral infections account for the majority of acutely inflamed throats. It is not always possible to differentiate bacterial from viral infections clinically. Throat swab culture and serum antibody levels may be required to make a definitive diagnosis. A brief description of some of the more important throat lesions follows.

Acute streptococcal tonsillitis and pharyngitis

Causal agent. β-Haemolytic streptococcus.

Clinical features consist of a sore throat, dysphagia and high temperature. The tongue is furred and there is oral fetor. Cervical lymph nodes are enlarged and tender. The patient is fevered and may have headache and earache. The tonsils and palate are red and swollen and there may also be spotty exudate on the tonsils (follicular type). Later exudate may become confluent (exudative type).

Diagnosis may be confirmed by the presence of neutrophil leucocytosis in the peripheral blood and by isolation of streptococci from a throat swab.

Treatment. (a) Penicillin, (b) aspirin gargles.

Notes
1. *Scarlet fever.* This essentially consists of streptococcal tonsillitis with the added feature of a skin rash produced by a streptococcal toxin.
2. *Peritonsillar abscess* (quinsy). This results from the spread of infection from the tonsils into the surrounding tissues. Pus collects behind the tonsil forming an abscess which often requires incision. Quinsy is not common in children.
3. *Ludwig's angina.* Cellulitis of the sublingual and submaxillary spaces of the floor of the mouth and neck pushes the tongue

upwards and may obstruct the airway. Treatment includes large doses of antibiotics. Drainage and sometimes tracheostomy are required.
4. *Other rare complications of streptococcal sore throat* include glomerulonephritis and acute rheumatic fever.

Diphtheria

Causal agent. Corynebacterium diphtheriae.

Clinical features. Diphtheria is now rare in Britain as a result of effective immunization campaigns. The commonest type affects the fauces where the local lesion takes the form of a thin translucent membrane which may spread from the tonsils to the palate, uvula and pharynx. As the organisms multiply in the local lesion they produce a powerful toxin which damages many tissues. The toxin causes the general symptoms of the disease.

Diagnosis. Diphtheria is diagnosed by culture of the organism from the local lesion.

Treatment. Diphtheria anti-toxin must be given along with penicillin therapy. Erythromycin is also effective in the treatment of the disease.

Viral infection of the throat and pharynx
Almost any of the respiratory viruses may be associated with an acutely inflamed throat. The adeno group of viruses are a common cause of acute pharyngitis, particularly in children and young adults. The A group of Coxsackie viruses may cause acute pharyngitis associated with vesicle formation on the soft palate and fauces. In children, in addition to mouth ulcers, Coxsackie virus may also cause blisters on the palms of the hands and on the soles of the feet (hand, foot and mouth disease).

Infectious mononucleosis (glandular fever)

Causal agent. Epstein–barr virus.

Clinical features. This is a common condition in older children and young adults. In the angiose form of the disease the patients present with sore throat, enlarged lymph nodes and fever. The tonsils may be covered by thick whitish exudate which may mimic diphtheria. There are often petechial haemorrhages on the palate. Other features of the disease include a maculo-papular rash, abnormal liver function tests and occasionally frank jaundice. Splenomegaly also occurs.

Diagnosis can be confirmed by finding atypical mononuclear cells in a blood film. Most cases have a positive serological test (Paul–Bunnell test). Glandular fever may occur in epidemics with a definite pattern of oral transmission.

Treatment. Antibiotic therapy is not indicated in confirmed cases.

Note. Patients with infectious mononucleosis very frequently develop an allergy to ampicillin and related drugs. These antibiotics should not therefore be prescribed for throat infections.

Herpes simplex mouth infections

Clinical features. The primary infection with herpes simplex virus type I usually occurs in early childhood and is manifested by ulcerative stomatitis. Affected children develop shallow painful ulcers on the buccal mucosa and tongue. The child is usually febrile, very miserable and refuses to eat or drink. The condition is self-limiting and the ulcers usually heal in about ten days.

Treatment. Consists of oral hygiene and correction of dehydration if this is present. Very severe infections may justify treatment with the anti-viral drug acyclovir.

Candidosis (thrush)

Clinical features. Infection with the fungus *Candida albicans* often follows the used of broad-spectrum antibiotics which kill the normal mouth flora and allow fungal super-infection. It also occurs in children and in the debilitated. Patients on steroid therapy and those who are immune-suppressed either by drugs or disease are particularly susceptible to 'thrush'. White plaques appear on the mucous membranes of the mouth, throat and tongue. Rarely spread to the lungs and gut occurs.

Diagnosis is confirmed by observing the fungi in a smear from the lesions and by the culture of the organisms.

Treatment. Local applications of an anti-fungal drug such as nystatin, miconazole, econazole or amphotericin usually clears infection rapidly. Antibiotic therapy should be stopped if possible.

Chapter 25

Acute (necrotizing) ulcerative gingivitis or Vincent's angina

Organisms. Vincent's organisms (coarse spirochaetes and fusiform bacilli).

Clinical features. An infectious condition affecting the gums, which become inflamed and spongy and bleed readily, or the tonsils. Tonsillar involvement is usually unilateral. There may be either a thick yellowish membrane on the tonsil or an ulcer with a dirty sloughing base and high edges. An offensive oral fetor is always present.

Diagnosis. Organisms are seen in large numbers in a smear taken from the lesion.

Treatment. 1. Penicillin and metronidazole are both effective in clearing the lesions. 2. Hydrogen peroxide mouth washes may be used.

Note. Eating and drinking utensils should be isolated and boiled.

Recurrent oral ulceration
Recurrent mouth ulcers, whilst extremely common, are on the whole trivial and most are not associated with systemic disease. The commonest form of recurring ulcers are aphthae.

These cause considerable distress and on occasion difficulty in eating. They may occur singly or in small groups. The cause of aphthous ulcers is unknown. A number of organisms, both bacterial and viral, have been suggested but conclusive evidence is lacking. Many patients have circulatory antibodies to oral mucosa. This finding may put the condition into the category of an autoimmune disease, but about 10% of cases have an underlying disorder, such as anaemia of almost any cause.

Treatment of aphthous ulcers remains unsatisfactory. Topical steroids applied early may be of benefit.

The differential diagnosis of recurrent oral ulceration includes various mucocutaneous syndromes—Behçet's syndrome particularly may present with recurrent painful mouth ulcers.

Disorders of the blood
Patients suffering from agranulocytosis (lack of neutrophil poly- morphs in the blood), aplastic anaemia (marrow failure) and acute

leukaemia may present initially with a sore throat and mouth. There may be ulcero-membranous lesions on the tonsils or pharynx and the gums may be infected and bleeding. Aplastic anaemia and agranulocytosis may represent iatrogenic illness related to the use of certain drugs or cytotoxic agents.

Treatment
Aplastic anaemia and agranulocytosis
(a) Stop any drug which could be causing the condition.
(b) Treat the throat infection.
(c) Blood transfusion as necessary.

Leukaemia.
(a) Treat throat infection.
(b) Induce remission of the disease.

Trauma to throat or pharynx
The possibility that an unusual lesion of the palate, throat or pharynx could be the result of trauma should always be kept in mind. Injury with objects such as pencils, toys and feeding bottles is not uncommon in children and at any age the throat may be traumatized by foreign bodies in food (fish bones, etc.).

26   Fitness for surgery and anaesthesia

Pre-operative assessment

The majority of dental procedures are performed in dental surgeries and a smaller number in local authority clinics. Local anaesthesia is the method of choice and the need for general anaesthesia has steadily reduced. The scope of local anaesthesia has been broadened by the use of intravenous sedation with drugs like diazepam or midazolam. Low concentrations of nitrous oxide (30%) in oxygen can also supplement local anaesthesia, the technique being called *relative* analgesia.

Indications for general anaesthesia

General anaesthesia must be justified. This group includes young children requiring multiple extractions, and of local anaesthetic patients exhibiting true hypersensitivity to the vascular absorption of local anaesthetic or to the adrenaline which it may contain. Acute local infection renders local anaesthesia less effective and risks spreading that infection. Often the mentally or physically handicapped cannot co-operate and require a general anaesthetic for conservation work and exodontia, as do some emotionally labile patients who can be weaned on to local anaesthesia later, helped by intravenous sedation or relative analgesia. Oral surgical procedures like removal of impacted wisdom teeth, excision of dental cysts and all major surgery like mandibular-osteotomy, tumour excision and major trauma require general anaesthesia.

Types of general anaesthesia

Induction of anaesthesia is usually by inhalation of nitrous oxide, oxygen and halothane in the young and by intravenous methohexitone (1.5 mg/kg) in older patients. Nasotracheal intubation when indicated can be achieved by deepening halothane anaesthesia or by intravenous injection of the short-acting depolarizing muscle relaxant, suxamethonium (1 mg/kg). Maintenance of anaesthesia is with halothane 0.5–1.5% and a minimum of oxygen 30% with nitrous oxide 70%. Halothane is a potent agent capable of producing vasodilatation, myocardial depression and cardiac arrhythmias, particularly during bone work in the mouth. The recently introduced inhalation agents enflurane and its isomer, isoflurane, are less liable to produce cardiac arrhythmias.

Local anaesthesia may be supplemented by the use of intravenous drugs like diazepam (0.15–0.3 mg/kg) or midazolam (0.07 mg/kg), the patient being kept conscious and cooperative throughout. The anaesthetist must be fully prepared to deal with cardiovascular problems, respiratory depression or apnoea, while maintenance of a clear airway is essential to the safety of this technique.

Patient selection for anaesthesia
It is vital that patients presenting for general anaesthesia, sedation and local anaesthesia are carefully selected and the decision made whether to operate in the dental practice, clinic or hospital. Clearly, major oral surgery and patients with serious medical problems require hospital care. Specialist clinics can provide facilities for many of the emotionally upset and physically and mentally handicapped. Life-threatening airway problems like severe trismus or oedema of the floor of the mouth must be treated in hospital.

Initially a questionnaire regarding medical history provides a screen. Questions to be answered on a No/Yes/Details basis include:

Specific disorders
   Hypertension,
   Diabetes,
   Jaundice,
   Asthma,
   Heart-attacks,
   Tuberculosis,
   Pregnancy,
   Problems associated with previous anaesthesia,
   Death in family associated with anaesthesia,
   Present illnesses other than presenting complaint,
   Recent or present drug therapy,

Allergies,
Other.

Symptoms or signs suggesting cardiovascular and respiratory disease
Effort tolerance impaired,
Breathlessness,
Nocturnal dyspnoea,
Ankle swelling,
Angina,
Palpitations,
Fainting or dizzy spells,
Cough,
Sputum,
Recent acute infections,
Smoking,
Wheezing.

Other
Liver disease,
Kidney disease,
Excess alcohol.

Physical examination of the otherwise fit patient in the dental surgery is usually brief and includes observation, palpation of pulse, measurement of blood pressure and auscultation of the chest.

Patients with significant medical problems require to be fully investigated and to be on optimum therapy prior to anaesthesia.

Cardiac disease
Cardiac failure untreated before operation carries a high mortality rate, therefore diagnosis and treatment are essential. Serum electrolytes must be checked because of the relationship between heart failure, diuretic therapy, hypokalaemia, digoxin and cardiac arrhythmias.

Ischaemic heart disease also carries a significant mortality rate after major surgery. Timing of operation in relation to a recent myocardial infarction is vital as the risks to re-infarction are greatest within the first three months. Ideally operation should be delayed until after the sixth month. The anaesthetist must be aware of current drug therapy like beta-adrenoceptor blockade with drugs like metoprolol or atenolol, and calcium channel blockade with nifedipine because of interactions with the inhalation anaesthetic agents. Unstable angina is a contraindication to general anaesthesia. A current electrocardiogram must be available.

Uncontrolled hypertension must be investigated and treated because it presents a threat to the myocardium during and after surgery. Tracheal intubation can cause a marked rise in arterial blood pressure. Treatment with cardiac and anti-hypertensive drugs should be maintained throughout the peri-operative period.

Congenital heart disease and acquired valvular heart disease must be fully assessed. Patients requiring major heart surgery often present for dental treatment first. Prophylactic antibiotic therapy is recommended for the prevention of bacterial endocarditis, e.g amoxycillin 2.0 g single oral dose one hour before dental work (1.5 g for children under 1) followed by three further doses of 500 mg at 6 hourly intervals. For patients allergic to penicillin, erythromycin 1.0 g should be given instead (0.5 g for children under 10). Gentamicin 1.5 mg/kg body weight intramuscularly or intravenously is added to ampicillin 2.0 g 30 min before the procedure when the patient has a prosthetic valve or a history of bacterial endocarditis, followed by 1.0 g amoxycillin orally six hours later (p.239). Antibiotic prophylaxis is not required for patients who have had coronary artery bypass surgery by itself.

Patients with artificial heart valves and on anticoagulant therapy can discontinue this two days before surgery, but require careful supervision, keeping the thrombotest less than 25%.

Respiratory disease
Integrity of the patient's airway during any anaesthetic procedure, whether under general anaesthesia, intravenous sedation, relative analgesia or local anaesthesia, is fundamental to safety.

Investigation and treatment of any medical condition compromising the respiratory tract is important and will also contribute to a reduction of post-operative pulmonary complications.

General anaesthesia should be avoided in the presence of acute upper respiratory tract infection because of the problems created by excess secretions. Acute bronchitis and pneumonia are contraindications to general anaesthesia. Chronic bronchitis and emphysema often produce secretions, fits of coughing and bronchospasm. Anaesthesia must be delayed until the patient has had the benefit of chest physiotherapy, bronchodilator therapy and antibiotics if indicated. Asthmatic patients who have been free of recent attacks and whose chest is clear on examination can be handled safely by the correct choice of anaesthetic agents. Chest X-ray is necessary for assessment of acute change or up-dating the progress of chronic disease.

Rib fractures, pneumothorax and pleural effusion may accompany major trauma and a chest X-ray is mandatory. If respiratory failure is supected arterial blood gas analysis is indicated.

Anaemia

Oxygen is transported to the tissues in combination with haemoglobin. A small volume only is dissolved in plasma. Reduction of the amount of haemoglobin, perhaps by haemorrhage, reduces the oxygen carrying capacity of blood and reduces the safety margin should a problem like respiratory obstruction occur during anaesthesia. A full blood count is desirable for in-patient surgery. Surgery is usually deferred when haemoglobin levels fall below 10 g/dl and corrective therapy is instituted. Whole blood or packed red cells should not be given in the 24 hours before surgery, unless to treat acute blood loss, because transfusion results in an initial reduction in 2,3-diphospho-glycerate (2-3DPG) inside the red cell which interferes with release of oxygen to the tissues. Blood must be grouped and held or cross-matched for major oral surgical procedures.

Sickle cell anaemia is the most common of the haemoglobinopathies. There is a risk of haemolysis and multiple infarction following minor hypoxia or hypercarbia in the homozygous type (SS). General anaes-thesia should be avoided if possible. The heterozygous type (AS) of sickle cell trait requires severe hypoxia to produce red cell sickling. It is essential to screen all West Indian and African patients for these abnormal haemoglobins.

Thalassaemia syndromes are the result of a relative failure of haemoglobin synthesis and are most common among Asian and Mediterranean races. A severe hypochromic anaemia can result, with bone marrow hypertrophy and mandibular overgrowth which may make tracheal intubation difficult.

Coagulation disorders (p.82)

A variety of disorders may cause excessive bleeding in children. Haemophilia A is due to synthesis of abnormal Factor VIII. Factor IX (Haemophilia B) is called Christmas disease and von Willebrand's disease is also due to low Factor VIII. The risk of bleeding varies with the patient and the extent of surgery. Cryoprecipitate or Factor VIII concentrate may be given intravenously just prior to operation in those with haemophilia A, but the physician in charge of the haemophiliac's care or the nearest haemophilia centre should always be consulted first.

Thrombocytopenia may be idiopathic or accompany leukaemia. Young patients with the latter present for dental treatment, and as with the previous disorders, close involvement with the haematologist and the blood transfusion service is vital.

Close supervision of cardiac patients on anticoagulant therapy has been mentioned already.

Hepatic disease
Reduced production of prothrombin increases the risk of haemorrhage and vitamin K may be required pre-operatively.

Altered levels of the enzyme pseudocholinesterase render patients with severe liver disease very sensitive to suxamethonium. The toxicity of local anaesthetic agents is increased in severe liver diseases.

Should a patient with jaundice require general anaesthesia full liver function tests must be available. The date of any previous exposure to halothane must be stated as re-exposure to halothane within about three months runs the risk of a hypersensitivity reaction to halothane. Agents like enflurane or isoflurane can be substituted. Patients with a history of hepatitis must have a serological test performed as a check for the presence of the virus A (Australia antigen) and virus B.

Renal failure
Severe renal disease is often accompanied by a marked anaemia, haemoglobin levels of 5 g/dl being not uncommon. Alterations in serum electrolytes, particularly potassium, will affect the use of suxamethonium. Recent haemodialysis may affect the circulating blood volume and cause cardiovascular problems during anaesthesia. Preparation of patients with severe renal disease requires a full blood count and recent serum electrolyte values.

Diabetes

Non insulin-dependent patients on oral hypoglycaemic agents of the sulphonylurea group (chlorpropamide, glibenclamide) or biguanide group (phenformin, metformin) can be managed by discontinuing their medication at least 24 hours before surgery. Chlorpropamide's effect may last for 6 hours. *The greatest hazard during anaesthesia is hypoglycaemia and blood sugar levels must be monitored before, during and after surgery* by using simple diagnostic aids like BM Stix or Gluko-chek.

Insulin-dependent. For relatively minor procedures under general anaesthesia the insulin-dependent diabetic should be transferred to short-acting Actrapid (neutral) insulin. The morning dose may be omitted or, preferably, half of the usual dose of insulin given plus intravenous infusion of dextrose and the blood sugar checked regularly (p.136). Early resumption of normal diet can be accompanied by the relevant dose of Actrapid insulin.

Major surgical procedures under general anaesthesia require management with an insulin–glucose–potassium infusion. The amount of insulin infused is dependent on the blood sugar levels, which are followed at least two-hourly.

Adrenal insufficiency

Patients with adrenal hypofunction like Addison's disease are treated with hormone replacement therapy. Adrenal steroids like hydrocortisone are also of value in the treatment of a variety of other conditions including arthritis, asthma, allergic states and skin conditions.

For non-major procedures, patients on steroid supplementation should have their normal regime pre-operatively and hydrocortisone 25 mg intravenously. Major procedures require their usual therapy pre-operatively, plus hydrocortisone 25 mg i.v. during induction of anaesthesia and hydrocortisone 100 mg/24 hour by infusion until resumption of oral feeding. This low dose regime should provide adequate protection against hypotensive collapse.

Pregnancy

Operative procedures should be avoided during the first three months of pregnancy. The risk of spontaneous abortion is not generally high, but any intervention could be blamed for this occurrence. After seven months general anaesthesia should be avoided because of the hazards of respiratory embarassment and aspiration of gastric contents.

Disease of the nervous system

Cerebral palsy is the principal cause of crippling handicap in children. Intravenous sedation or general anaesthesia may be necessary to allow dental treatment because of uncoordinated and involuntary movements. In severe cases, marked skeletal deformities may make tracheal intubation awkward.

Epilepsy and convulsions are controlled by anticonvulsant drugs like phenytoin, sodium valproate and carbamezepine. Methohexitone is contraindicated for epileptic patients and thiopentone may be used for intravenous induction.

Diazepam 0.2 to 0.3 mg/kg intravenously is the drug of choice for the control of status epilepticus. Hypoxia must be avoided and careful observation is needed in the post-operative period.

Hydrocephalus. A ventriculo-peritoneal or atrial shunt is usually used to aid the flow of cerebrospinal fluid. These patients require antibiotic cover for surgery and should be treated in hospital.

Down's syndrome. Nearly half of all children with this syndrome (trisomy 21) have a cardiac lesion, often an atrial or ventricular septal defect, or Fallot's tetralogy, and antibiotic cover may be necessary. Though mentally retarded (there is a wide range of intelligence), these children are usually cooperative and not difficult to handle. Airways difficulties can arise due to the size of the tongue, while nasal catarrh and nasal bone abnormalities, and micrognathia, can present problems.

Dystrophia myotonica can occur in children and adults. This is an inherited disease characterized by myotonia associated with muscle weakness and wasting. Cardiac muscle may be involved too.

Problems can arise from respiratory depression from quite modest doses of drugs like diazepam, or the inhalation agents. The response to suxamethonium may be abnormal causing prolonged muscle contracture thus making the patient impossible to ventilate or intubate. Dysrhythmias and reduction of cardiac output may arise if myocardial depressant drugs are used when cardiomyopathy is present.

Index

302 *Index*

Uropathy, obstructive 212
Uveo-parotid fever 113

Vaccines 107–9
Vagus nerve, lesions 176
Varicella 200
Vascular disease
  peripheral 33
    smoking and 245
  see also Cerebrovascular disease
Vasodilators 41, 47
Vasovagal attack 9
Venereal diseases 252–40
Ventilation, artificial 50
Verapamil 32
Vertigo 280
Vesicle, definition 255
Vincent's angina 290
Viridans streptococci endocarditis 37
  treatment 38
Virus infections *see* Infections, viral
Vision, ageing and 204
Vitamin deficiencies 166–9
Vitamin A deficiency 166
Vitamin B deficiencies 167–8
Vitamin B_{12} deficiency 78–9
Vitamin C deficiency 168
Vitamin D
  deficiency 151, 166
  intoxication 154
Vitamin K deficiency 167
Von Willebrand's disease 82, 84

Warfarin 2, 3, 42, 86
  dental extractions, in patients receiving 88
  interactions with other drugs 87
Weal, definition 255
Wernicke's encephalopathy 167
Wheeze 53, 62, 67
Whooping cough 197
Wounds
  dehiscence 5
  healing 20
    causes of delay 21

  nutrition and 6
infection
  clinical presentation 22
  management 22
traumatic
  infection 20
  management 20

X-ray therapy 96
Xanthine bronchodilators 65
Xerostomia 112

Z-plasty 23
Zygoma, fracture 19